Praise for

The Thousand Mile Stare
and Gary Reiswig

"Gary Reiswig, the last man standing in a generation ravaged by inherited, early onset Alzheimer's Disease, tells a family history like no other. His unique memoir explores the best hope that modern medical science offers to anyone facing the ultimate identity theft of Alzheimer's—especially Reiswig's own nieces and nephews, who are just now reaching the age when their destiny may express itself."

— DAVA SOBEL, *New York Times* bestselling author of *Galileo's Daughter, Longitude,* and *The Planets*

"A powerfully moving and extraordinary story told with a courageous heart."

—Lisa Genova, author of the *New York Times* bestselling novel *Still Alice*

"This powerful narrative tells not only the story of the many lives devastated by Alzheimer's, but also the tremendous courage of the people in this family who participated in research study with hope as the only tangible benefit. Someday, when a treatment is developed, and methods derived to prevent Alzheimer's disease, scientists will take the credit. But it is really the thousands of volunteers that courageously participate in research that make breakthroughs possible. Read this book."

—Gerard D. Schellenberg, Ph.D., Department of Pathology and Laboratory Medicine University of Pennsylvania School of Medicine

"Gary has given me a face, as he has to his family by writing this book. I like to believe that Gary's cousin Chuck and I are LIVING with Alzheimer's not dying from it. This book keeps our fires alive and I am grateful to him and his family for continuing to fight the war on Alzheimer's."

—Kris Bakowski, diagnosed with early onset Alzheimer's at age 46

"Gary Reiswig compassionately brings us close to the fear and suffering that he and his family endure as Alzheimer's plays itself out in each successive generation. . . . Studies suggest that the chances of developing the disease by age 85 is now close to 50/50. Thus, there is something very personal for us all in *The Thousand Mile Stare*. We all stand to face the Reiswigs' 50/50 dilemma unless we act to change the trajectory of this pending public health crisis."

—**William E. Klunk, M.D., Ph.D., recipient of the 2008 Potamkin Prize for Research in Pick's, Alzheimer's and Related Diseases**

"This is a must-read book for the early onset people and also for the caregivers. I am a person with early onset and I had trouble putting the book down."

—**Mary Lockhart, diagnosed with early onset Alzheimer's at age 55**

"Alzheimer's disease struck members of Gary Reiswig's family in the prime of their lives. *The Thousand Mile Stare* provides a riveting account of his family's quest to understand and cope with this devastating disease."

—**Marie Pasinski, M.D., Neurologist, Harvard Medical School, Massachusetts General Hospital**

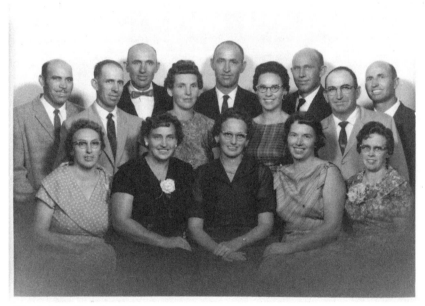

The Reiswig Family, 1959

The
THOUSAND
MILE STARE

The

THOUSAND
MILE STARE

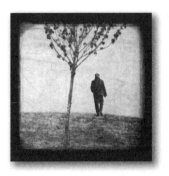

*One Family's Journey through the Struggle
and Science of Alzheimer's*

GARY REISWIG

n_b_

NICHOLAS BREALEY
PUBLISHING

BOSTON • LONDON

This edition first published by Nicholas Brealey Publishing in 2010.

20 Park Plaza, Suite 1115A   3-5 Spafield Street, Clerkenwell
Boston, MA 02116, USA   London, EC1R 4QB, UK
Tel: + 617-523-3801   Tel: +44-(0)-207-239-0360
Fax: + 617-523-3708   Fax: +44-(0)-207-239-0370
www.nicholasbrealey.com

Printed in the United States of America

14 13 12 11 10   1 2 3 4 5

ISBN: 978-1-85788-536-1

Library of Congress Cataloging-in-Publication Data
Reiswig, Gary.
    The thousand mile stare : one family's journey through the struggle and science of Alzheimer's / Gary Reiswig.
      p. cm.
    1. Alzheimer's disease—Popular works.   I. Title.
    RC523.2.R45 2009
    616.8'31—dc22

                               2009044674

Contents

Contents

This book is dedicated to my Aunt Ester May, and my cousin, Chuck, two courageous people of different generations. Without them, there would have been no book. Due to their courage, our story is one of hope, not despair.

Acknowledgments

M y immediate family—my wife and children—contributed substantially with ideas and support in the writing of this book, especially Julie Hanson Reiswig, my daughter-in-law and my researcher, who used her considerable savvy to uncover kernels of information I could not have included without her help.

Gary Miner, and his wife, Linda, supplied material from their Alzheimer archives and valuable memories about the work in the seventies and eighties with Aunt Ester and my extended family. One sentence cannot possibly encapsulate the sacrifices and contributions they made to Alzheimer's research on behalf of our family.

Gary Reiness in Portland, Oregon, helped me understand and simplify the complex scientific issues I needed to explain in the narrative.

It is not adequate to merely say "thank you" to Doctors Thomas Bird and Gerard Schellenberg and the rest of those on the University of Washington research team who dedicated ten years of their lives to help find the rarest gene, PS2, which affects our family. Hopefully, you will understand that this book is also a small measure of thanks.

Many of my relatives sent thoughts and ideas. Some may be surprised their contributions have not been included in the book. Unfortunately, through the editing process, some material fell to the floor, as is often the case when bringing a book to fruition. However, much of the lost material will appear on the book's web site (www.thethousandmilestare.com). My dedicated editors at Nicholas Brealey Publishing deserve a lot of credit for sticking with this book; also my sincere thank you to my writing group led by Hope Harris for countless insights.

Elizabeth Kaplan, my agent, kept the myriad needs of the writer in her mind even as she concentrated on our wish to get the work published.

I have kept the need of and wish for privacy within my extended family uppermost in my mind with every word I have written. For the sake of privacy, sometimes I have avoided using names. In other cases where the narrative seems to need an identifying name, I have supplied pseudonyms. I hope my dear loved ones will forgive me if they don't particularly care for their new names or the names of their family members.

To my dear sister and brother: I wish I had been more attentive when you were alive because I miss you terribly now that you are gone.

To the others who deserve mention and credit for their support and contributions to this book, thank you.

Foreword

I have worked with the Reiswig family for nearly twenty-five years and know many of the individuals described in this book. Their story is tragic and compelling. Surprisingly, they are not alone. They suffer from a mutation in one of three genes known to cause early onset familial Alzheimer's Disease. Symptoms of memory loss and confusion begin in the forties and fifties, the prime of life, just as experienced by Mr. Reiswig's relatives. Each child of an affected parent is at fifty percent risk of inheriting the abnormal gene and also developing the disease. More than 200 such families have been recognized worldwide. And this number is dwarfed by the four million persons with Alzheimer's living in the United States with the much more common (but less well understood) later onset form of the disease. Fortunately, the type of Alzheimer's disease occurring in the general population is not strictly genetic with such a high risk to relatives as occurs in the Reiswig family. However, these rare genetic families appear to be a good biological model of the more common form of Alzheimer's disease. Information resulting from scientific studies of families such as this has provided and will continue to provide important insights into the biology of the disease. Although present medication is modestly effective at best, better treatments and preventive therapies are sorely needed. Partly because of knowledge gleaned from families such as the Reiswigs, I am convinced that these better treatments and preventatives will be found. It is only a matter of time, effort, and resources. No one can predict when this time will come. We all hope it will be sooner rather than later so that future generations of this family will be spared from continuing the sad story reported here.

Thomas D. Bird, M.D.
Professor, Neurology and Medical Genetics
University of Washington
VA Puget Sound Health Care System
Seattle, Washington

Huntoon Crossing

❧

T wo men left the Tulsa Airport in
Oklahoma and headed southwest on the Turner Turnpike. It was
late March, 1986. The trees and grass were trying to turn green,
but the two men paid little attention to the landscape, focused as
they were on the task before them. They were after blood—my
family's blood.

These men—one a neurologist, Thomas Bird of Seattle,
Washington, the other, a clinical researcher, Gary Miner of Tulsa—
were out to help, not harm. My family needed that help. For years,
we had kept information about dotty parents, loopy aunts, and
childish uncles to ourselves. After our blood was drawn, these
strangers, and countless others, would examine our DNA under a
microscope exposing problems that had been kept within the family
for generations, opening our family secrets to the outside world.

To some members of my family, this prospect was terrifying.
But nothing could be as frightening as what we'd already been
through.

❧

I n the early winter of 1936, my grandparents, John and Mollie, and one of
my uncles, Otto, a lanky basketball star at his high school, left their home
in the Bluemound community of the Oklahoma Panhandle and headed to
Booker, Texas, the nearest town where they could sell eggs and cream at the
local produce market. They were luckier than many of their neighbors

1

because they had extra produce to sell, and could purchase other supplies with the proceeds.

Long before they crossed into Texas, they could see the tin Huntoon grain elevator, the tallest structure within miles, where freight trains had stopped to load grain during the good years following World War I. As they bounced their way south over the country road—hardly more than a track—the only other man-made structures on this barren plain came within sight. There was the flat Huntoon store, which had opened in 1929, just as the Depression hit, then closed soon after for lack of business, and the cross-like warning sign erected by the Atchison, Topeka, and Santa Fe Railroad. The black and white sign, and the rusty ribbon of track that angled southwest to northeast, stood in sharp contrast to a few inches of snow that had fallen the night before, bringing the farmers a quarter-inch of moisture and a large dose of hope.

There was not a tree or even a tumbleweed to obscure my grandfather's view of the wide-open prairie as he drove his small cattle truck over the Texas state line. Just before the railroad track, the road inclined slightly. As the truck passed over the track, an eastbound train struck it on the passenger side. The impact killed my grandmother and severely injured my uncle, who spent the next five months in a hospital bed in Perryton, Texas. My grandfather needed several stitches to sew up a gash in his head.

At the time their mother died, six of my grandparents' fourteen children, ranging in age from five to seventeen, were still living at home. Several more moved back home when they didn't have jobs. That was a lot of mouths to feed. The Dust Bowl gripped the panhandles of both Texas and Oklahoma; drought and choking dust prevented crops from growing. But both of my grandparents were from hardy German stock and knew how to survive in difficult times. Their ancestors had migrated from Germany to Russia, where they learned how to farm the steppes, a barren landscape not that dissimilar from the Oklahoma Panhandle and the rest of the United States Great Plains, an area called "The Great American Desert" less than a century earlier.

To feed the milk cows, the family pulled the thistles that grew in the fencerows. The chickens ate table scraps, weed seeds, and, in the summer, the infernal grasshoppers. So the family managed to get by.

It was a miracle that all fourteen siblings in my father's family were born alive and healthy and survived. My mother grew up just down the road from my father's family; two of her siblings died in infancy. Most other families in the area had similar stories—babies born too fragile to survive in the middle of a drought. Dust pneumonia and malnutrition were common, not only in the vulnerable young ones, but also among the adults.

All the children in my dad's family appeared to be vigorously healthy. His generation obeyed God's command to Adam and Eve in the Garden of Eden, "Be fruitful and multiply," although the barren countryside resembled the Garden of Eden not one iota. Still, a new generation was on its way despite the worst of hard times.

My grandmother's life had been cut short before she became a grandmother, a status highly valued in a family-centered culture. The first two grandchildren, my cousin Carolea and my sister, were born soon after she died. Both girls looked like their grandmother, which brought the family a little bit of comfort.

I was nine or ten when I found out how my grandmother died. My dad and his family never talked about it, even though they got together for a potluck dinner several times a year at one sibling's house or another. They ate fried chicken, drank iced tea, and visited while they played pitch, rook, or horseshoes. But they didn't talk about their mother and dad. My mother was the one who told my sister and me how Grandma died.

Not long after she told us, our parents drove us to Perryton for a checkup with the family doctor. Driving west on Texas State Highway 15, we passed through Booker, where my grandparents were heading the day of their accident. A mile or two out of town the road bent south, parallel to the railroad track. We passed the Huntoon elevator. A few houses and one or two machine shops were clustered on the other side of the road, and the store that closed during the Depression had reopened. On the west side of town, Mother pointed and said, "There, that's where the accident happened that killed your grandmother."

My father, who was driving the black four-door 1947 Plymouth, the only vehicle he ever bought new, did not turn his head to look, but my sister and I crowded over to the window in the backseat. There was nothing to see except the crossing sign where the country road rose up and crossed the railroad tracks. From that day on, when we passed the crossing, I'd always stare, trying to imagine what happened. What possibly could have caused my granddad to drive in front of a train?

When I was in high school, my girlfriend and I sometimes went to Perryton to go roller-skating. Once we made the trip on a summer evening, when the sky was still light. After we passed through Huntoon, I turned on the country road. I had a spooky feeling as we approached the crossing sign. After looking both ways, I drove over the railroad tracks. Then I turned around and drove over the tracks again. I tried to imagine what my grandparents and my uncle were talking about when the train hit them. Or, were they sitting silently, lost in their own thoughts until the impact?

Neither my granddad nor my uncle could explain how the crash happened. In addition to severe internal injuries and many broken bones, my uncle suffered amnesia as a result of the crash. After he recovered consciousness, he couldn't remember anything about what happened immediately before or after the accident. My grandfather was mute, in shock, grief-stricken. In any case, I don't think he *knew* how he got into the path of an oncoming train. No one pressed him for answers. No one wanted to hear the horrible details. But still, everyone had questions.

Before the accident, the family was aware that my grandfather had become a little forgetful, but they assumed he was distracted by worries about providing for them and keeping the farm going during hard times. Maybe his distraction had contributed to the accident. Another theory: The passenger side window of the truck was broken, and Granddad had replaced the glass with a piece of cardboard. Perhaps, despite the wide-open view at the crossing—where train smoke could be seen for miles—this broken window obstructed Granddad's vision.

My dad and his siblings embraced the broken-window theory. But silent contradictions kept them pondering. *Couldn't see the train? For Christ's sake, you could see that train for miles through the front windshield! The road ran straight south, and the track angled southwest. A slight glance to the right was all you needed.*

The period following the accident was terribly difficult for Granddad and the children because Grandma was the family's anchor. But they stayed together. Some of the older unmarried daughters came home to help their younger siblings. They reared my youngest uncle and aunts, who were only five, eight, ten, and twelve when their mother was killed. My uncle, Otto, who was seventeen at the time of the accident, recovered, graduated from high school, and took over management of the farm because Granddad no longer could do the job.

In the years following the accident, Granddad's condition declined, more mentally than physically. His doctor prescribed a raw egg in a glass of warm goat's milk. Whether this helped Granddad is up for debate. But watching their dad throw back his head and gulp down his breakfast, gagging and retching, did give his children a moment of amusement in what was otherwise an endless stretch of bleak days as the drought continued. Day after day, the relentless panhandle wind lifted dust clouds that filtered the sun's weak rays. On holidays, the girls livened up the house with taffy pulls and made dark chocolate fudge and fluffy white divinity with nuts.

After the Japanese bombed Pearl Harbor, the boys who were old enough and unmarried went into the service. My uncle Otto had recovered almost completely from the accident, except for a slightly crooked arm because the doctors didn't get the bones set perfectly. For a time, the draft board avoided drafting him because they knew he was needed at home. In 1942, following harvest, he was notified to report for induction. He became a driver for the Army's medical service in Europe.

My aunts left the Bluemound homestead also. One became a secretary in the City of Wichita garbage department. One became a teacher. Two others got married. Although the drought had broken and the Dust Bowl ended, the damage was done; Granddad had to give up the rented farm. Granddad and my youngest uncle, who was still in grade school, stayed at the homes of the married children.

When Granddad stayed with us, nights were difficult for my parents because Granddad woke up and wandered. They were vigilant day and night as if they were the parents of an infant. When I was five they taught me to tell time on my father's pocket watch, and had me take my grandfather out for walks. Mother attached the fob and chain to my overall suspenders to make sure I didn't lose it. "Watch out for the electric fence so he doesn't touch it, and stay away from prairie dog holes so he doesn't trip. Don't come back until the big hand is here," they instructed me.

I held Granddad's hand while I led him across the road toward a pond with a willow tree growing beside it. To me, Granddad was a mystery. I didn't know why he was so quiet. My other grandfather, Granddad Gregory, was a great talker and tease, lively and fun to be around. But this granddad didn't talk at all. He hardly seemed to notice me. Sometimes he stopped and stared, with a glazed, faraway look. Years later, my cousin Chuck saw that same look on his mother's face; he termed it "the thousand mile stare." This was my first experience with Alzheimer's disease, but I didn't know it. No one did.

Chapter One

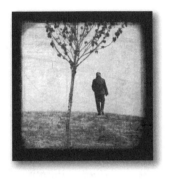

FROM HESSE
TO HUNTOON

"The first symptom the 51-year-old woman showed was the idea that she was jealous of her husband. Soon she developed a rapid loss of memory. She was disoriented in her home, carried things from one place to another and hid them, and sometimes she thought somebody was trying to kill her and started to cry loudly.

In the institution her behavior showed all the signs of complete helplessness. She is completely disoriented in time and space. Sometimes she says that she does not understand anything and that everything is strange to her. Sometimes she greets the attending physician like company and asks to be excused for not having completed the household chores, sometimes she protests loudly that he intends to cut her, or she rebukes him vehemently with expressions which imply that she suspects him of dishonorable *intentions. Then again she is completely delirious, drags around her bedding, calls her husband and daughter and seems to suffer from auditory hallucinations. . . .*

As the illness progressed . . . the imbecility of the patient increased in general. Her death occurred after four and a half years of illness. At the end, the patient was lying in bed in a fetal position completely pathetic, incontinent. . . .

Specimens which were prepared according to Bielschowsky's silver method show very striking changes of the neurofibrils. Inside of a cell which appears to be quite normal, one or several fibrils can be distinguished by their unique thickness and capacity for impregnation. . . . Finally, the nucleus and the cell itself disintegrate and only a tangle of fibrils indicates the place where a neuron was previously located."

—An English Translation of Alois Alzheimer's 1907 Paper, "Uber eine eigenartige Erkankung der Hirnrinde", Clinical Anatomy 8:429-431 (1995). Translated by Stelzmann, Schnitzlein, and Murtagh.

*

In 1901, Alois Alzheimer, a neuropathologist in Frankfurt, Germany, examined a fifty-one-year-old woman, Frau Auguste Deter, a patient in the asylum for the mentally ill and epileptics where Dr. Alzheimer was the senior physician.

Before confining her to the asylum, Frau Deter's family was in despair. Frau D no longer could care for herself, but she rejected the family's attempts to help her. When she left her house unattended, she wandered the streets of Frankfurt, getting lost, cursing at strangers, looking unkempt and deranged. She screamed at her husband in public, accusing him of infidelity, and accused her doctors of raping her.

When Dr. Alzheimer examined her, he found that, in addition to other symptoms, she had severe short-term memory loss. He called her condition, "presenile dementia." There was no effective treatment. She died nearly five years later.

By then, Alzheimer had left Frankfurt and was working in Munich with doctors Emil Kraepelin and Franz Nissl. Alzheimer obtained permission from Frau D's family to examine her brain, and it was shipped to Munich. He used a silver staining technique to study her brain tissue under a microscope. On November 3, 1906, at a meeting of German physicians, Alzheimer presented a three-page paper describing the amyloid protein plaques and neurofibrillary tangles in Frau D's brain. The plaques and tangles he observed and reported on comprise the clinical description of Alzheimer's disease.

Today, there is hardly a person who does not know the name Alzheimer. Alzheimer's disease has pulled up alongside cancer as one of the two most dreaded diseases in the western world.

*

In 1766, 140 years before Alzheimer presented his short paper in Frankfurt, my ancestor Johannes Reiswig, his wife, Catherine, and their eight-year-old son, George, packed up their few belongings. They had always lived in the Hessian countryside near Frankfurt, where Alzheimer would practice a few generations later. They were poor Lutheran farmers. With several thousand other German peasants, they departed Hesse for a year-long trip to Russia. This was not a vacation, but a migration to what they hoped would be a better life.

Four years earlier, Catherine the Great, a former German princess turned ruler of the Russian empire, had issued a manifesto inviting people to immigrate to her country and settle on the steppes, the remote plains of the Russian frontier. Catherine had designed the manifesto so it would be most appealing to her fellow Germans—sturdy farmers living in states where princes paid more attention to their own pleasure than to the needs of their subjects. Skilled farmers could help Catherine bring a new level of prosperity and stability to an unoccupied part of her adopted country.

When he read the manifesto and made the decision to move, Johannes Reiswig was fifty-seven or fifty-eight—some twenty years older than his wife. Johannes probably had been married before. He may have had sons that had been conscripted by the princes to fight for one mercenary army or another. This could be why he and his wife Catherine decided to take their young son on the risky journey to Russia. In addition to free land, the Russian empress had promised the farmers exemption from military service.

The Reiswigs made it safely to Russia in 1767 and settled in the village of Walter (named after its first German mayor). Johannes died during the first winter. We don't know what happened to Catherine—she may have remarried or raised young George on her own. But we know George survived, married, and had a son named Adam George. Adam George had a son named George. And George had a son named Jacob, who was my great-great grandfather.

Jacob and his second wife, Anna, had four sons. The oldest, Christian, my great-grandfather, was born in 1860. In 1871, the Russians began a program of integrating the German colonists into the Russian social order. In that process, the Germans lost one protection Catherine had granted in perpetuity: exemption from military service. The Russians began drafting the Germans' sons into the Russian army as soon as they turned twenty-one. The prospect of having Christian fight and kill for the Russian army—a most *un*-Christian act, in their view—may have helped spur Jacob and Anna Reiswig to gather up their belongings and leave Walter in the spring of 1878, bound for the United States. Christian was seventeen when the family began their journey.

In the United States, the Reiswigs expected to find not only protection from forced military service, but also available land. President Lincoln had signed the Homestead Act of 1862, granting any settler 160 acres of land, if the settler agreed to improve his allotment and live on it for a minimum of five years.

After Jacob, Anna, and their sons cleared immigration on Ellis Island, they headed for Marion County, Kansas, the final stop on the Atchison,

Topeka, and Sante Fe Railroad, and the town where some German Mennonites, who had left Russia a few years earlier, had settled.

Christian went to work as a farm hand. In his early twenties, he married Mollie Heinrich. My grandfather, John, was born in 1883, the first of five children. A few years after Granddad's birth, the family moved from Kansas to Oklahoma, settling with other Germans near the town of Kiel, named after a town in Germany. That town is now named "Loyal," because during World War I the town's name was changed, a blatant attempt by the Germans, still laden with heavy accents, to convince the local Ku Klux Klan they were loyal to the United States.

Mollie Heinrich, my great-grandmother, had died at age thirty-five. We don't know why she died so young. Christian died in 1903 at the age of forty-three. Some family reports indicate that Christian was senile by then. Christian's second wife, Lena Brown, and their infant daughter, died the same year as Christian. We don't know the cause of the family's demise.

The graves of Jacob and Anna, and Christian and Mollie, lie adjacent to one another in a Seventh Day Adventist Cemetery a few miles west of the town that is today still called Loyal, Oklahoma. When they reached America, why the Reiswig family converted from Lutheranism to Seventh Day Adventism is open for speculation. The change might have had much to do with becoming American, giving up a religion from Europe, and embracing a vigorous religious movement that grew out of the impulse to tame and convert the prairie into farmland and homes.

My grandfather was fourteen years old when his mother, Mollie, died; his youngest brother, Sam, was just four. Six years later they lost their father.

My grandfather then went west to the Oklahoma panhandle. Sam remained behind, and stayed in Kingfisher County for the rest of his life.

My dad and I visited Uncle Sam several times when I was a child. Sam's farm stretched out in gentle, undulating hills, verdant wheat waving in the wind. One time I asked my dad why Uncle Sam's wheat looked so much better than ours. "They get more rain, son," he replied. Later I learned that Sam lived east of the 98th meridian; we lived west, on the high plains, where it was preordained that the annual rainfall would average less than twenty inches.

It was the familiar search for wheat land that sent my grandfather west to the panhandle, where the topography and the climatic conditions nearly replicated the conditions of the Russian steppes. It was there, beyond the 98th meridian in No Man's Land, that my dad's oldest sister was born in 1906, the year Frau Auguste Deter died back in Frankfurt and Dr. Alzheimer looked at slices of her brain under a microscope and found plaques and tangles. In 1907, the year Oklahoma became a state, Dr. Alzheimer published his paper about Frau Deter's brain, giving his clinical description of what would be called Alzheimer's disease. In 1908, my grandmother gave birth to another child; a third was born in 1909. My father was born in 1911. Ten more followed, the last one arrived just as the Dust Bowl began in 1930.

It was there, in the midst of the Dust Bowl, that my grandfather, grandmother, and uncle set out to deliver their produce to the creamery in Booker, Texas. Granddad, as he had done scores of times before, slid behind the steering wheel of the small cattle truck, and headed toward the Huntoon crossing.

Chapter Two

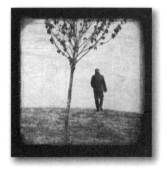

THE FAMILY PROBLEM

My *family's involvement in research with the University of Colorado Department of Neurology began in the 1970's, and ended in the early 1980's because there was no funding. After less than a decade, we were research orphans. Then my Aunt Ester May was invited by U.S. senators from Oklahoma to testify before a Senate committee in Washington about our family's disease. As a result of those hearings, and many efforts on the part of many individuals, the Congress recognized the severity of the Alzheimer's epidemic looming as the current post-World War II generation reached maturity. The Congress, through the National Institute of Health (NIH), then funded the Alzheimer's Disease Research Centers across the country, and what was termed the "War on Alzheimer's" began.*

Soon after the first ADRCs were funded, my Aunt Ester— who had pushed, cajoled, and prayed our family into our research

involvement—assisted Dr. Gary Miner and his wife, Linda, set up a
meeting in my hometown church. With their own money and some
grants, Gary and Linda had started a foundation to promote
Alzheimer's research, and they persuaded some of the best
researchers in the world to journey to this remote Oklahoma pan-
handle town to share the research they were doing with each other
and to meet with our family and hear our story. Among those
researchers who attended was Thomas Bird, M.D., a neurologist
with the newly funded Alzheimer's Disease Research Center in
Seattle, Washington. The Seattle center had designed a study of
familial early onset Alzheimer's disease, with the express purpose of
looking for the gene that causes it. This was the real beginning of
the real research, the search for the early onset Alzheimer's disease
(EOAD) gene that runs in our family.

I n 1962, when I was about to turn twenty-three, I was living with my wife
and two sons in a small town East of Indianapolis. I was working as a youth
minister at the Fortville Christian Church and was attending graduate school
at Lincoln Christian Seminary in central Illinois, some 200 miles from our
home. After more than a year on a very difficult schedule, I was offered a position as minister of a church only ten miles from the seminary. The church
promised that I could divide my time between the ministry and my studies. I
accepted the offer, and we moved to Illinois. That was around the time my
mother called to tell me Dad was "becoming quite a handful."

She and Dad had gone to town on a Friday, which they often did, to
shop and take care of business. Mom got out of the car at Denzil's Grocery, and
Dad drove on down Main Street to the bank. They agreed to meet at the store
when he finished banking. When he didn't show up, Mother left the bagged
groceries at Denzil's and walked from the store to the bank. The car was
parked in front. An employee told her Dad had been in and left an hour ago.

Mother walked both sides of Main Street, ducking into stores she thought he might have gone into, but she couldn't find him. She walked a block west to the county courthouse, and he wasn't there. On the way out of the courthouse, she saw the sheriff sitting in his patrol car. She asked him if he'd seen Dad. "I saw him walkin' north, out of town. I asked him if he needed a lift, but he said no, he was meetin' you. I figured you two were having a picnic up in the sand hills," the sheriff said, as if worried that Mother might think he was neglecting his duties.

The keys were in the car, so Mother drove north toward the sand hills. She found Dad walking fast along the highway, nearly half way to Forgan, the next town. He told her he knew he was supposed to meet her but he couldn't remember where, so he decided to go home, figuring that's where she was. "But you're walking in the wrong direction," she told him. "And you left the car parked in front of the bank."

Meanwhile, on their farm, my Uncle George and Aunt Ester May faced similar problems. They had married shortly after Uncle George returned from World War II. Ester had lost her first husband on the last day of the fighting on Okinawa. After George and Ester May married, he farmed and she taught school. Then Uncle George, influenced by his wife, decided to become a preacher and a farmer just like Ester May's father had been.

In the late 1950's, shortly after my uncle graduated from Midwest Christian College and they returned to the farm, Ester May began noticing changes. He could no longer repair simple mechanical breakdowns, and there were major delays in the farm work. The furrows he plowed weren't straight. He parked the farm machinery at random; before, everything had been parked in neat rows. The farm began to look unkempt, disheveled. If he drove any distance from the farm, he sometimes got lost and had to call Ester May to help him get home. If he walked out the back door at home, he was fine. If he went out the front door, a door they seldom used, he might get lost. He had trouble performing his duties at church, fumbling for words when he was called on to pray. When he was asked to be a guest preacher, he wrote out his sermons word for word and read them.

Ester May was smart and had the courage of a fighter pilot. And, unlike my mother, she took a confrontational approach to life. Ester May drove my uncle to doctor after doctor, trying to find an explanation for his behavior. One doctor believed Uncle George's troubles stemmed from trauma suffered during the war—what we now call post-traumatic stress syndrome. Another doctor thought he had a thyroid problem. Another accused Ester May of being the problem. By being so forceful and opinionated, he suggested, she had undermined her husband's confidence. My mother, and others in the family, did not like the way Ester May was dealing with the problem, making it so public, and Mother might have agreed with that diagnosis had she not been facing the same problems with Dad.

Ester May caught on to what the rest of the family couldn't see, or chose not to see. Ester May not only saw it, she also talked about it. She said out loud to the family, her husband's problem was not merely an individual problem, it was a family problem. All we had to do was look around us.

🌿

Dad's oldest sister, Pearl, the last Seventh Day Adventist in our immediate family, was more advanced in her symptoms than were Dad and my Uncle George. Pearl had to quit her job in Wichita because she could no longer do the work. Her husband, Bob, struggled to work and take care of her. One evening he came home and found she had put ice trays in the stove instead of the freezer. Then Pearl physically attacked him because there was no ice. Uncle Bob retired early from the Wichita, Kansas, Department of Refuse so he could care for Aunt Pearl full time.

Dad's sister Alta, who was younger than Dad but older than Uncle George, was the first in our family to get divorced. At first, the family blamed

16

her ex-husband. But eventually it became clear that the split wasn't entirely his fault. Aunt Alta was very difficult to live with. She was so disorganized and forgetful that her son, the same age as my younger brother, had to move out and live with relatives who could better care for him. He lived with us for a school year.

So that made four siblings with similar symptoms.

Everyone except Ester May seemed to have forgotten about Granddad. No one talked about the fact that Granddad was "a little forgetful" before the accident at the train tracks. The family assumed that Granddad's silence and detachment after the accident were due solely to grief. No one, except Ester May, linked the symptoms of my dad's generation—forgetfulness, disorganization, difficulty performing mechanical tasks that once had been routine—to the accident at the Huntoon crossing.

*

Faye Meyers, a physician who practiced in Oklahoma City, was one of the few doctors in the United States who had, by the late 1950's and early 1960's, studied a seemingly rare degenerative disease called Alzheimer's. After Ester May spoke with dozens of doctors who gave her all kinds of diagnoses and prescriptions for my uncle's problems, a local doctor who had heard of Dr. Meyers suggested Ester May take George for an interview.

By that time, Mother was desperate for answers, too. She knew that she and Dad couldn't continue to operate the farm. She had been acting as his foreman, and his parent, for several years. Each day she got him up and dressed and told him what he was supposed to do, and then she checked on him several times an hour. She was exhausted from the effort to keep him going, weary from the strain.

At Ester May's suggestion (this was one of the few times Mother ever took her sister-in-law seriously), Mother made an appointment with Dr. Meyers. Fearing the worst, Mother asked me to come home from Illinois and accompany them to the examination. It was then we heard the words *Alzheimer's disease* for the first time. Dr. Meyers helped us recognize, and start to come to terms with, the family problem.

My mother geared up for the long siege that Dr. Meyers warned her Alzheimer's would bring. She turned the farm over to my sister and her husband, and helped Dad resign from the church board. She and Dad moved to town. Mother organized Dad's closet and drawers, and invented a system of notes and reminders. But Mother said nothing about Dad's condition, or her own suffering, to anyone. If someone asked her why they had moved to town, she said, "It was time for the next generation to take over the work. We're just going to enjoy ourselves."

Uncle George could no longer work either. Ester May taught school to support the family. When she got a better job offer, she moved the family to Kansas. Unlike Mother, Ester May talked to everyone about my uncle's condition, how difficult he was to care for, and how dangerous it was to leave him home alone. Over and over again, she emphasized the need to involve the whole family in what was a family problem.

When Ester May heard of a doctor with a new theory or treatment, she'd make an appointment. Some family members claimed she carted George to so many doctors because she wanted one of them to tell her to put him in an institution.

Ester May thought there ought to be a family research center to study our "Alzheimer's problem." She said she'd donate land where lakeside cottages could be built for afflicted family members, who could live there with their caregivers. Doctors could visit them and do research onsite.

Ester May was never popular in our family; even before the Alzheimer's problem came to the fore, she'd always been one to talk about taboo subjects. But now—as she pushed the family to be open about the disease and get involved in a research program—her openness and determination were less welcome than ever.

Mother said, "I wish she'd stop talking about Alzheimer's. It does no good to talk about it. We just have to live with it." When my family and I were home visiting my parents, Mother asked me to tell Ester May not to talk about the disease in front of Dad. "Just because he has it doesn't mean he has to hear about it," Mother said.

Most of the family avoided Ester May as much as possible, but she would not be avoided. She marched right in, said her "howdy," and spoke her mind. For the most part, my generation listened and took her words to heart. She was the one we talked to when we had concerns and questions.

*

Moving to town didn't make Dad happy. Mother saw it in his body language. He had no energy and slumped when he walked. He sat around watching television, which drove Mother nuts. She tried giving him odd jobs; he'd start them but then get lost before anything was completed. Nothing in his surroundings was familiar except some tools Mother had brought from the farm. So she had unfinished flowerbeds and a half-made garden bench.

Mother decided they had to move back to the farm. She hired Uncle Otto, who was a carpenter, to build a small house near my sister's home. While my uncle was working on the house, Mother drove Dad out to the construction site so he could help. Or, perhaps more accurately, my uncle babysat Dad while Mother went down to the farm to spend time with my sister. Mother came back up to the new house every hour or so to check on things. Uncle Otto was endlessly patient with Dad, and Dad started to feel better. He could still drive nails. Sometimes the nail went in the wrong place, but it went in.

Dad asked again and again whose house it was going to be. Both my uncle and Mother told him many times a day. He understood for a few minutes, and then he forgot. By the time the house was finished, Dad was so disoriented that he hardly realized the farm was just a half-mile over the hill.

That winter, my brother-in-law, Scott, took Dad along when he fed the cattle. Scott put the truck in first gear and climbed on the back to kick off the hay while Dad guided the truck, just as I had done for Dad when I was five. That was the highlight of his winter days. He did the job of a five-year-old. But it made living in the country a whole lot better than living in town.

Three years later, my office phone rang. I was the minister of Central Christian Church in Pittsburgh, Pennsylvania, near the University of Pittsburgh, where I was enrolled in a Ph.D. program. When I answered the phone, I heard a sharp intake of breath and I knew it was Mother. "Your dad's in the hospital," she said.

I caught the earliest flight I could arrange. While I drove with Mother to the hospital, she filled me in on Dad's condition. She told me his liver was failing. What an irony for a man who never took a drink. "He looks horrible," she said. "His face is yellow. Doctor Calhoon says there's not much to do. Just wait to see if he gets better or worse. He says it depends on what part of the brain is affected. Don't be surprised if he doesn't know you." She paused and then said, "I think it's better if he goes now. Do you think it's wrong to pray for him to die?"

When I got out of the car, Mother said, "I'm not coming in with you. I'll do some grocery shopping so we have something for supper and leave you and your dad alone for a while."

Weeds were growing through the cracks in the sidewalk, although it was only April. The door to Dad's room was open. Late-afternoon light filtered through a dirty window. His hair, what there was of it, was uncombed and stood up in disarray against the light. When he saw me, the look on his face changed. He either knew me, or he knew he should know me.

I pulled up a chair close to him. I put out my hand and, after pausing a few seconds, he lifted his to meet mine. His grip was strong, and we gave each other a firm, country handshake. Although he'd done little work for the past couple of years, his hand still felt calloused and rough. "Hello, Dad," I said. He smiled at me but remained tentative. I resisted the impulse to ask, "Do you know who I am?"

His face was jaundiced, more deeply lined than I remembered. I didn't know what to say. He tried to talk, but the words and syllables were jumbled. "It's okay, Dad," I said. "I've come to see you. Mom says you're having a rough time."

He laughed. The sound was deep, from the back of his throat, as if he were saying, "You don't know the half of it."

We sat for a while without saying anything. Then I tried to tell him things I thought he might be interested in. I told him my boys were playing T-ball. Then I thought, "given the arguments we'd had about me not doing the farm work so I could play baseball, he probably doesn't want to hear how I'm passing on my love of baseball to his grandsons." I told him how much I liked my classes at the university. "I've been reading western history books," I told him. "I remember when you showed me buffalo trails across our land. Remember? We were riding Lady and Dusty, getting the cows in." His eyes were focused—less cloudiness, more clarity.

"We should have kept her," he said. The sentence was clear; Dad sounded perfectly normal. I knew he was referring to the filly, Lady. We had sold her and kept her half brother, the gelding, Dusty, who wasn't worth a damn as a cow horse.

Finally, a hospital aide wheeled in a meal cart. I wondered if Dad could feed himself. As if on cue, Mother arrived. She took the fork and fed him. He ate everything. Nothing wrong with his appetite. It was obvious Mother had been feeding him for a long time.

After the meal cart was wheeled away, Mother said to me, "We should get you home and feed you. You look skinny." Dad tried to say something. After a few missed syllables, we understood. He wanted to go home, too. Mother told him Dr. Calhoon wanted him to stay, and he couldn't come with us. As she patted down the wisps of wild hair on his head, I got a lump in my throat I couldn't swallow. I didn't want to stay any longer, but I found it difficult to walk out of the room and leave him. He'd been dazed and confused when I first arrived, and then he'd become focused and lively. Now that we were leaving, he appeared frightened. I wondered if he was afraid to be left alone—afraid of dying. Afraid of dying alone.

Chapter Three

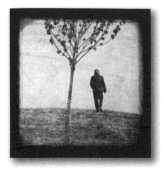

GENIUS OF
THE DUST

W*hen I was the minister of Central Christian Church in Pittsburgh, there was a college student, Gary Reiness, who was a part of my congregation. We have maintained contact with each other over the years. Eventually he became a professor of biology at Lewis & Clark, in Portland, Oregon. In February, 2008, when my family was visiting in Portland, we had dinner with Gary and his wife, Paulette. I told him I was writing this book, and I had a question: What causes a mutation in a gene? Following is his answer, which he later sent me in an email.*

The mechanism for copying DNA—which is required every time a cell divides, including the cells that give rise to eggs and sperm—is a bit imperfect and makes a mistake once out of every one to ten billion tries, according to most estimates. That sounds pretty good until you consider that all the genetic information in a human consists of about three billion nucleotide pairs (the basic building block of DNA), so each time a cell divides there's a risk that it will accumulate the alterations that we call mutations. If the actual error rate is one in a billion, then there are about three mistakes each time a cell divides, since the DNA synthesis machinery needs to make three billion decisions to copy the DNA. If the error rate is only one in ten billion, then that's still about one mistake in every three cell divisions. The main point is that the rate of such errors is very low, but it's more than zero.

Most of these mutations are either inconsequential (so-called silent mutations) or lethal, so the cell dies and doesn't pass on the mistake. Some can even be beneficial and improve a function or create a new function. The mutations that are problems are the ones that occur in gametes (reproductive cells, namely eggs or sperm) and that are both harmful and not immediately lethal, so that they can be passed on and cause damage to the next generation. This is the case with your family's mutation and many others that cause human health problems like cystic fibrosis and Huntington's disease, or more mundane effects like lactose intolerance or inability to roll the tongue. Mutations can also be induced by chemicals (mutagens) like those in tobacco smoke, formaldehyde, etc. and by radiation, including the ultraviolet radiation in sunlight, x-rays, etc. In that case the error rate would be higher. But even if you could avoid all radiation and only eat pure, uncooked food (some cooking generates mutagens) and breathe pristine air and drink pure water, you'd still accumulate mutations because of the imperfect DNA copying machinery. (Actually the machinery is very good, but no biochemical process has 100% accuracy, and in our case, the DNA copying accuracy is probably better than 99.999999%, but still not perfect.)

A s best as it can be explained, that's what happened to my family. A muta-tion occurred in an egg or a sperm at some point in our history. We don't know which ancestor this was. It might have been in the dark ages, the middle ages, or the industrial age, but from that ancestor forward the genetic makeup was in place so that each child of an affected parent has a fifty-fifty chance of inherit-ing the mutated gene that causes early onset Alzheimer's disease. All we know is: this occurred before my great-great-grandfather Jacob was born in Russia in 1837.

My mother and father were married in 1934, in the middle of the Dust Bowl. My dad had a job on the Schultz ranch, a combination cattle ranch and wheat farming operation in the Texas Panhandle. After the wedding, performed by a local justice of the peace, my parents went to Darrouzett, Texas, a small town about fifteen miles from the Schultz ranch. They posed in their wedding clothes near the local tourist attraction, the new steel bridge over Kiowa Creek. Then they had dinner with friends, mostly relatives, at the local cafe.

My sister once asked our parents if they went on a honeymoon after they got married. "Oh yes," Mother said, her voice brightening with the memory. "We went to Darrousett." She showed us the picture of her and Dad standing in their wedding clothes beside the bridge.

The Schultz family had assembled thousands of acres of land, gobbling up parcels from small owners who couldn't survive the panhandle's extreme condi-tions and either sold their property at bargain prices or lost it to the bank, which then offered it to the Schultzes. The Schultzes gave my mother a job cooking for the ranch hands. They also gave my parents a house to live in and paid them a hundred dollars a month, good wages for the time.

Less than two years after my parents were married, my Uncle Harvey came to tell them my grandmother had been killed at the Huntoon crossing. When I asked my mother about it, she said, "No one could believe it. We wore our wedding clothes to the funeral. Everyone sat around and didn't say anything. No one could understand how it happened."

My sister was born the next summer. Despite the drought, there was a decent harvest on the ranch that year. She arrived just as harvest ended, and Mother said it was a relief to go to the hospital and get off her swollen ankles for a few days. My sister had large, dark eyes like my dead grandmother. My dad's brothers and sisters noticed the family resemblance.

I was born two-and-a-half years later, in the tiny ranch house where my parents lived, in the middle of a howling blizzard with only my grandmother attending to my mother and me. My dad had left on horseback three days before to check cattle. Dad was gone for a week. He'd taken shelter in a line shack and escaped frostbite, but he couldn't save dozens of cattle that smothered or froze to death in the drifting snow.

My dad subscribed to *The Farmer Stockman* and every other farm magazine available. He read every article and ordered every free pamphlet about the newest farming methods, and he learned from working with the Schultzes. By the time I was two, my parents had saved some money. They purchased a section, 640 acres, of Dust Bowl–ravaged land in Beaver County, Oklahoma, fourteen miles from where they both had been born. They spent $640 of their savings for the ten percent down payment.

Before my dad tried to plant and harvest any grain from the tillable acreage, he had to stop the erosion that had depleted the rolling land. The native grass sod had been plowed under around 1910 to help meet the worldwide demand for wheat.

He borrowed more money from the bank, and hired a company with a road grader and a bulldozer to build terraces that would stop the erosion. Dad planted grass in the drainage areas, on the steepest parts where even terraces were ineffective, and on the hilltops where the topsoil had all blown away.

A year or two after he purchased the land, Dad and Artie Evans, a neighbor, bought an old Baldwin combine together. Dad kept it running with his innate mechanical skill. In the late forties, Artie bought a brand new self-propelled Massey Harris, and gave his half of the Baldwin to Dad on the condition that Dad would help maintain his new combine.

In 1950, it was so wet at harvest time that many farmers lost their wheat crop. Their machinery got mired in the mud and wheat stalks gave way and fell over. Dad and Artie planned to help each other with harvest. Artie's new combine, with a lighter body and wide tires, managed to cut without getting stuck. The heavy, lumbering old Baldwin, with thin wheels pulled by an M International Farmall tractor, got stuck before it was ten feet in the field.

Dad hooked on a second tractor. They both got stuck. Watching Artie sail over the muck with his lighter combine riding on wide tires gave Dad an idea. He drove to Amarillo, Texas, where there was an Army Air Corps base that had surplus airplane tires and bought two balloon tires. After half a day of work with the blowtorch and welder, he had them mounted on the combine. These huge wide tires rolled smoothly over the muddy places.

When other farmers, waiting to get in their wet fields, heard what Dad had done, they drove over to look. They stood around in their muddy overshoes, hands in their pockets, shaking their heads in disbelief. The combined circumference and width of the new tires put more surface on the wet soil to hold up the combine. Dad's knowledge of mechanical physics had solved the problem.

When harvest was over, Artie repeated over and over, "The man's a fucking goddamn genius. I tell you, a goddamned genius."

A year later, the climate was totally different. Beginning in early spring, the sun burned bright every day and the temperature climbed into the hundreds. The wheat planted the prior fall withered in the spring. The farmers waited for moisture so they could plant sudan, kafir corn, and milo, the spring crops that feed the cattle through the winter. When it didn't rain, many planted the seed anyhow, hoping against hope. But the seed lay in the dry soil and did not germinate.

Grasshoppers came, as they had in the 1930s, in clouds—like one of the plagues of Egypt—and ate the plants that sprouted in the low-lying, wet areas, and the leaves off the trees. Many farmers, knowing they had no way to get their livestock through the winter, took them to the sale barn. But the cattle looked thin, prices were low, and there were few buyers.

The preachers claimed we were in the final days that St. Paul had warned his young disciple, Timothy, about. *"This know also, that in the last days perilous times shall come."* Church attendance surged.

By this time, my dad had become an elder in our church. He prayed for rain along with everyone, but he also took action and explored alternatives.

Dad had been thinking about digging an irrigation well for a long time. Finally, he decided to do it. "We'll pump enough water to grow feed for a hundred head of cattle," he said. Mother was skeptical.

Bud, the county agent, was against the idea too. He gave Dad a report prepared by the federal government years ago, claiming that irrigation on the Great Plains was impossible. The source of water, the Ogallala aquifer, was too deep and too unreliable for irrigation.

But Dad was determined. He said there was a guy down near Darrouzett who could find water with a willow tree branch. The next day, Dad drove out to find him. Just before chore time, he returned. "Did you find the water witch?" Mom asked.

"Yep."

"Well?"

"He was drunk," Dad replied.

The next day, Dad walked over to the pond in the east pasture where I once had walked with my granddad. A substantial willow tree grew at the edge of the pond. He came back with a branch five feet long, with a fork on one end. Then he took off across the property.

A half hour later, he came back in the house. "I know where we're gonna dig the well," he said.

The site was near the large pond he had dug northwest of the house. He hired a well driller to dig a test hole. At 210 feet, the driller hit bedrock. Then he brought in the big rig. It would be the biggest well ever drilled in the county, 24 inches across.

The irrigation well was finished in a few weeks, paid for with money borrowed from the bank. When the engine started, a six-inch stream of water, more than 600 gallons a minute, flowed into the concrete tank Dad had poured, then out of the tank into a sluice that ran into the pond.

Bud was there when the first water came gushing out. He said he'd never seen anything like it; it seemed like a miracle. "But I'm a man of science, and I don't believe in miracles," he added.

I stood near my dad, looking out at the pond brimming with water. "Did you find this spot with the willow?" I asked him.

He chuckled and put his hand on my shoulder. "I realized it was better to pump the water out of the pond than directly from the well onto the fields," he said. "The pond is the same distance from all the fields we'll be irrigating, and the pond holds a lot of water. If the well motor stops, we can keep irrigating while repairs are made." He pulled me up against him, hugging me very tight. "You won't tell your mom, will you? I also have another idea, but it's a surprise."

He dug a swimming pool beside the pond, covered the bottom with sand and gravel, installed a diving board made from a bridge plank, and created a neighborhood recreational center.

Before, to picnic near water, we had to drive for miles. Now, with a constant supply of fresh water, our family and friends could spend Sunday afternoons swimming, fishing, and picnicking in and around a fresh body of water where once there had only been a muddy, cow piss–polluted puddle that might gag a catfish.

I watched the sparkling well water run down the sluice toward the pond that my dad had already stocked with perch, bass, and bluegills. Although I knew it was a sin to cuss, in my mind I echoed the words of Artie Evans from a couple of years before: "The man is a fucking goddamn genius. I'm telling you, a goddamned genius."

When I was nine, we went to the Boren Hereford Ranch to buy some cattle. Dad bought a bull calf that would be castrated for me to raise, fatten, and show at local fairs. He also purchased eight head of registered heifers, and a bull, on condition that I help him keep up with the paperwork required for registration. That was the part that appealed to me, selecting names for each new calf based on its lineage, like Devon Zato Heir, III. I loved the sound and rhythm of the names we selected.

The registered bull Dad bought would service the other beef cows we owned, in addition to the eight registered heifers, and, he hoped, would improve the quality of—and the profit from—all the calves we raised.

The non-registered cattle we owned had all been dehorned. We trained the horns of the registered animals to grow downward by attaching lead weights to them. Sometimes an animal would lose one weight, and we had to bring it in, herd it into a chute, and replace the missing weight to make sure the horns grew the same way on both sides. All this was more trouble than dehorning, but it was part of the package, like paperwork, when raising registered Herefords.

When the registered cows had calves, we selected the best of both the young heifers and bulls, kept them in the barn to fatten them, and trained them to compete at the county fairs with the stock of other farms and ranches. Competing for ribbons was my favorite part of farming. And the more blue ribbons our registered purebred animals won, the more money we could ask for our calves when we sold them.

Within two years, we had a dual beef operation going—selling registered breeding stock at premium prices to other farmers and ranchers who wanted to improve the quality of their herds, as well as the cow/calf operation from the unregistered herd. By the time we got the irrigation well, I had raised several show calves, and with the money from their sale, had purchased registered heifers. I was a minor partner with my dad in a small, but high quality, herd of purebred, registered Herefords.

With water flowing from the Ogallala aquifer onto the fields, we grew alfalfa south of the house, green pasture north of the house, and fodder for silage west of the house. The alfalfa and the silage were stored for use during the winter, and the cattle were run on the green pasture during the summer. This plan provided feed for the cattle from irrigated land year round.

Drought conditions had hung on, so other farmers' cattle were thin. But at the end of summer, our calves were slick and fat. We held the best ones over to feed and fatten for sale in the spring, when prices tended to be higher. But those we sold in the fall also brought premium prices because of their comparative quality.

By using the irrigated pasture, we gave the regular dry pasture a chance to recover from the strain of continued drought and constant grazing. The irrigation system made us feel immune to the whims of nature. Dad said, "I think I might buy a brand new truck." I went with him and we looked at the GMCs. I wanted him to have a new truck. He deserved something for himself, and it would be a measure of our success. In the end he resisted. "The old truck is fine," he told me on the way home.

The next spring, when the irrigated pasture was ready for cattle again, Dad told Mother he'd be away for two days and then, with no further explanation, simply disappeared. She and I were bewildered by his behavior; it wasn't like him to go off on his own, and he'd *never* done so without telling us where he was going. But we carried on, doing all the chores without him.

Two days later he returned, followed by two semi-trailer truckloads of thin, cheap, New Mexico cattle that had been running wild on sparse range, eating mostly mesquite and sagebrush. He planned to fatten them on our better grass and sell them in the fall. Since I considered myself a partner, I was surprised he hadn't asked me what I thought of the idea, or at least told me he was going to do it.

Dad unloaded the cattle in the east pasture. They were tall and skinny, with prominent hipbones and ribs showing beneath their rough, patchy skins. Within minutes, it was obvious Dad had bought nothing but trouble. These animals had not been dehorned; nor had their horns been trained downward. Used to a life of constant hunger, they'd learned to use their horns to get through fences so they could search for food. A three-strand barbed wire fence hardly fazed them, nor did the shock from a six-volt electric fence. They roamed the farm, and the countryside. We spend hours on horseback rounding them up, repairing the fences they destroyed. Mother and I were angry with Dad for the trouble he had brought us. But he remained his usual, steady, up-before-sunrise and to-bed-at-nightfall, self.

A dry southwest wind ushered in the summer; the temperature reached 110 degrees in June. The high temperatures toughened the grasses in the irrigated pasture and made the fodder more difficult to digest. By mid-summer, a third of the wild cattle had either died of bloat or had maggot-infested slits in their sides, where we'd cut them open to let out the gas and save their lives. In mid-July, we rounded up the ones that were still alive, drove them to the sale barn, and sold them.

Dad and I sat on the plank risers of the sale barn surrounded by other farmers and ranchers. Drovers with electric prods pushed our cattle into the sale ring. On the open range, these animals had a kind of wild, majestic self-determination I'd learned to respect, despite the immeasurable grief they'd caused us during their brief stay on the farm. Beneath the lights and whirring fans of the sale barn, as drovers climbed the fence to get out of the way of their slashing horns, these cattle looked deranged and malformed. The auctioneer begged the buyers to get involved and raise the bid. "These cattle look a little rough," he said, "but they're good for more than fertilizer." No one believed him. They sold for pennies a pound to an out-of-town buyer. Artie, sitting on the other side of my dad, said, "That's the dog food buyer."

On the way home, Dad tried to make a joke. Forcing a grin, he said, "Good thing I didn't buy that new truck." I felt horrible for him, but also angry. I didn't say it, but I thought, "Next time, talk your ideas over with someone first." I was fourteen years old and getting cocky. And I was starting to lose confidence in my dad.

I knew other kids my age got angry with their parents, but I wondered if my feelings were different. I was changing, but he seemed to be changing, too. I watched him from the corner of my eye as he drove toward home. He had opened the top few buttons of his shirt to cool off after enduring the close heat of the sale barn. The brown of his neck ended abruptly where the white of his shoulder sloped away. His head drooped forward. Shadows deepened the lines on his tired face. Neither of us said another word during the trip home from the sale barn.

We nicknamed one of our registered heifers Bronc because she wasn't tame like the others. Bronc had all the markings and conformation of a Hereford, but temperamentally she was a throwback to an undomesticated primitive breed.

That winter after Bronc had her calf, a bull, Dad asked me to bring her and the baby to the corral and vaccinate the calf for scours and check to make sure his testicles were descended.

I fed Bronc some grain to distract her, but it didn't work. When I grabbed her baby and threw him on the ground, Bronc attacked me and pinned me to the wooden boards of the corral. She jabbed at me with her horns, which we had trained downward with horn weights. Dad heard me screaming, picked up a loose fence post, and fought her off. I was shaken, but unhurt. Dad was scared and upset. "Leaving the horns on these cattle was a mistake. I'm gonna dehorn them," he said. His words cut into the pit of my stomach like the blade of a rusty knife.

I defended Bronc. I told him I was fine, that she couldn't hurt me because of the way we had trained her horns. "She was just being a good mother," I insisted. "I don't want her horns cut off." Dad listened to me, but Bronc continued to be a problem.

Later that winter, we were feeding the cattle silage and Bronc attacked one of the dehorned, unregistered cows. It's the kind of thing that happens all the time in a herd of cattle, but it threw Dad into a rage. He cussed, damning Bronc with language he hadn't used since he joined the church and became an elder. I had never seen him so angry. His rage seemed out of perspective, unbalanced.

"I'm gonna cut off their horns," he said again. Again, I begged him not to. I made the same arguments. The horns are harmless the way we train them. Dehorning them won't keep them from attacking each other. If he was concerned about Bronc, he could dehorn her, or sell her. We shouldn't dehorn every registered Hereford we owned because of the actions of one.

Their value as purebred cattle would be diminished. He listened, but didn't seem to be persuaded.

When I stepped off the school bus a few days later, the farm was quiet, with none of the usual sounds of animals and machinery. "What's going on?" I asked Mother. "Where's Dad?"

She told me he was down at the barn. "Artie and Harvey have been here all day helping him do something with the cattle," she told me. I went down to the corral to see for myself. There were horns everywhere, with white hair and bone still attached. And blood—blood on the chute and corral boards, thick and slippery on the ground. I stood on the second highest of the corral boards so I could see into the pasture. The dehorned registered purebreds stood with their heads near the ground, eyelids half-closed. A black smear of tar to stop the bleeding covered the raw place where their horns had been, but trickles blood broke through the tar and ran down their necks. I put my hand up to the side of my head. It must be like having your ears cut off, I thought. I estimated the value of the registered cattle had dropped by at least a third with this violent, useless act. I had never felt so helpless and ineffectual.

Back in the house, Mother tried to comfort me. "He hasn't been the same since the trouble with those New Mexico cattle," she said.

"I can't figure out what got into him," I said. "It was like the devil possessed him. Cutting the horns off those registered cows was crazy."

A few days later, my dad, Artie Evans, and I were squatting outside on the lawn talking about wheat prices. Mother never let Artie in the house because he chewed tobacco. Dad went inside to help Mother with a shelf that had come down. Usually Artie would take an opportunity like that to tell a dirty joke or ask me about my sex life. This time Artie's pale eyes wandered to the hillside across the road where the dehorned cattle were grazing. He spat a brown stream of juice on the lawn. "That sure is a sorry lookin' bunch of registered Herefords," he said. Artie was a smart rascal. I realized he knew, as well as I knew, something was going wrong with Dad.

Chapter Four

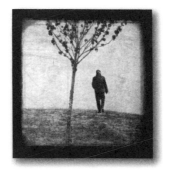

CONFRONTATIONS

I doubt I would have given my brain much thought if it were not for Alzheimer's disease, and what I saw it doing to the brains of people I loved. After Dad was diagnosed with Alzheimer's, I found myself reading about brains, listening to programs that talked about brains, and I started to marvel. I found out my brain is about the size of my two fists if I clench them and press them together. It weighs about three pounds. In my brain, there are a hundred billion neurons linked to each other in one hundred trillion pathways. This part always made me think of the Bible, where it says, "The stars in the heavens cannot be numbered." My brain makes up the most complicated system that exists anywhere, including the universe. My brain controls everything I do; I eat and digest, experience all the smells, tastes, and textures of the process; I move, play tennis, write, read; I breathe, and the brain controls all that happens *with the air I take in and expel; I am seduced by one person and repulsed by another because of my brain. I could go on and on.*

Now when I think of my father, I don't dwell so much on the fact that he lost his mind, his ability to think clearly and reasonably as the plaques and tangles accumulated without our knowledge — instead I marvel that he was such a remarkable man with a wonderful brain who accomplished so much in a tough environment. When Dad's brain was working, it had worked very well indeed.

I n late winter when I was eleven or twelve, it was just getting light when my dad and I headed out to the barn to do chores. The March wind, unusually strong so early in the day, howled through the bare branches of the elms Dad had planted as a windbreak. We were halfway to the barn when he stopped. "Listen," he said.

"What?"

"It's spinning too fast. The windmill." We walked over to the windmill, which stood beside our well house. It was taller than the average windmill; Dad built it higher to rise above the windbreak he'd planted, so the trees wouldn't cut down on the amount of wind, and, consequently, the amount of water the windmill pumped. I looked up through the center of the windmill's barn-red tower. The propeller spun so fast that the blades were blurred and the rods were clanking in the pipe.

As I looked up at the spinning blades, Dad looked down. He bent over and picked up a metal nut nearly two inches in diameter. "The brake — that's what happened. This has to be fixed before the wind picks up more."

I was familiar with windmills because Dad always made a point of showing me what he was doing when he worked on things. I had helped him assemble the windmill across the road in the east pasture. We used wire stretchers to hoist the mechanism to the top of that tower. I was on the ground pulling while my dad was on the tower putting the components together.

The windmill's tail keeps the blades of the propeller turned properly into the wind so that when the wind strikes the blades at the correct angle the propeller spins. However, if the wind is too strong, the propeller may spin dangerously fast. If this happens, centrifugal force triggers a mechanism called the brake. The brake causes the propeller to stop following the tail and turn sideways, away from the wind, so it slows down. Dad was holding a nut that fell off the brake, so the brake no longer worked.

"You go up and fix it and I'll start the chores," Dad said.

I thought he must be joking. When I was a younger kid, I'd played on top of the storage tank that rested on the well house, but I'd never been on the platform of the windmill. We kids never dared to climb it. It was higher than the peak of the barn.

"Naw, that's all right," I said. "You go ahead and fix it. I'll start milking." I expected him to grin and agree.

"If you can go all the way over to Clearlake for baseball practice, you can fix a broken windmill," Dad shouted back at me. Maybe he was raising his voice because of the wind, but he was definitely not joking.

His comment about baseball didn't come out of left field. Baseball was a sore point between us. For the last year or two twice a week I went AWOL from the farm because of it. I drove ten miles over back roads to Clearlake, where Pop Dinwiddie, a former Texas League baseball player, ran a general store and coached a group of ragtag country kids in unmatched hand-me-down baseball suits. Our team was the scourge of the flashier, better financed, teams in the surrounding towns. We had won every game we played last year.

Dad didn't object to my going all that way for practice. He objected to my love of the game, to the fact it was more important to me than farming.

To get out of fixing the windmill, all I had to do was turn around, walk back to the house, and tell Mother what Dad was asking me to do. She'd never agree to send me up the windmill tower on a windy morning to fix a broken brake. She would stop this.

But instead of relying on Mother again, I said to Dad, "I'm not sure how to fix it."

"See that piece of iron that starts at the tip of the tower and extends out, sort of like a horizontal 'v'? That controls the brake. Get hold of it and tie it to the tower with some wire. That will stop the blades from spinning. Find the chain. At the end of the chain is the bolt this nut fits on. That bolt fits through the end of the 'v.' I'll get you some wrenches. Tighten up the nut, unfasten the brake, and we're set. Simple, huh?"

I walked to the shop with him. He handed me the wrenches I needed and a piece of baling wire. I walked back to the windmill. He went to the barn.

Hand over hand, I climbed the windmill tower. The tower shook in the wind as the propeller spun. The whole contraption felt much less sturdy than it looked from below. I looked down for a moment. Feeling a little dizzy, I looked back toward the spinning propeller, and then I closed my eyes and caught my breath.

Just as I was about to grab hold of the triangular piece of iron to stop the propeller, the wind changed direction, and the tail swept over me. If I hadn't seen it coming, it would have caught me in the side and knocked me off the tower. I was scared.

A disturbing thought came into my mind: *He's down there in the safety of the barn, where, at worst, he might get kicked by a cow. I'm up here on a shaky tower in a shifting wind, and I could get killed.* Now I was not just afraid but also angry.

I decided to stay flat on the platform for a while and try to figure things out. As I lay there looking up into the gray sky, the wind shifted back, and the tail swept over my face again. There was no way to get the job done without standing up. While I tied the brake down to stop the propeller, somehow I'd also have to watch the tail so I could duck in case the wind changed again. Then I'd have to slip the bolt through the brake and tighten the nut.

With one eye on the tail, I stood up. I wired the brake to the tower, and the propeller stopped turning. Next, I slipped the bolt through the hole in the 'v,' screwed on the nut, and tightened it. I took off the baling wire and dropped flat down on the platform.

Back on the ground, I cranked the brake on and off several times to make sure it held. This gave my knees time to stop shaking.

Mother was surprised when I came in the house. "Quick chores!" she said.

"The brake on the windmill was broken. I fixed it. He can do the chores by himself."

She looked at me. "Let me get this straight. You got up on the windmill in this wind and fixed it while he started the milking?"

"Yep." I felt a little guilty, as if I were telling on a playmate who did something naughty.

"Sometimes I think that man's going crazy," Mother said.

The summer before my senior year of high school, I was pitching for the town American Legion team, as well as a team in Perryton, Texas. People knew me as the farm kid who could make his fastball rise left or sink right just by changing his grip on the ball, like a real major-league pitcher.

One day that summer, I was plowing wheat stubble in the field east of the house. Tall roiling black clouds arose in the southwest, and I knew they were coming my way. I had one terrace to finish. If I left the field, I'd have to come back out and finish when the clouds passed. I figured they weren't the kind that produced a full-blown storm—probably just a brief windy spell with some rain, and a little thunder. I wanted to finish the plowing because I was pitching that night against a good team in Liberal, Kansas.

My coach had told me there'd be a major-league scout at our game that night. This might be my chance to become a major league ballplayer, a dream I had harbored for several years, despite the fact I had publicly promised in front of our preacher, his daughters, and hundreds of others attending Christian service camp, to become a minister.

I still had a little plowing left to go when the wind whipped up and changed directions. A few hailstones, nearly the size of baseballs, fell around me. A lightning bolt struck the pasture a few hundred yards away, sending a little plume of smoke into the air.

I stopped the tractor and put up the umbrella. Hail never lasted more than a minute or two. The lightning was my major concern. With the umbrella up, the tractor could attract a lightning bolt. Whack! Bright light. A loud crackling behind me. A blast of wind, as if from an explosion. I didn't see where it hit, but it was close. Wham! A blinding flash to my left, no farther than a pop fly to right field. Then I saw the rain coming, sheets of it, swept sideways by the wind. By the time I unhitched the tractor and uncoupled the hydraulic hose, I was drenched.

I put the tractor in high gear and headed toward the house. The rain was so heavy I couldn't see ten feet in front of me. I drove along the fence to keep my sense of direction. Claps of thunder and flashes of lightning came one after the other, crackling so loudly my ears rang. Yellow and blue electricity danced along the barbed wire.

Now I understood. God had no intention of sending me to the major leagues. That was my own selfish plan. I had promised him I'd be a preacher. I wouldn't back out. "I promise I'll be a preacher. Just let me get to the house," I said. "Just let me get home." And the Lord granted my prayer.

That night, after the storm had passed, I gave up six runs, and we lost the game with a New York Yankees scout in the stands. My major league aspirations were over. I was going to be a preacher.

Two years after Dad installed the airplane tires on the old Baldwin combine so he could pull it in a muddy field, he bought a slightly used Massy Harris self-propelled combine, the same model Artie Evans owned. Every winter he took both machines apart and checked them. He told me it was important to know how to repair your own machinery, even if I was going to be a preacher. So on weekends I helped him.

I wanted to learn mechanics, but I was more interested in learning about cars than combines. Taking apart a combine was boring, brutal, backbreaking, grease-smeared, knuckle-bleeding work. But to Dad, the random pattern of chains, sprockets, belt wheels, shafts, cotter pins, and screening pans—all washed with gasoline so bright spots of wear or the smallest hairline cracks were visible, then laid out on a canvas—was far more beautiful than any painting.

My help was more perfunctory than competent. He'd ask me to put the "what-you-may-call-it" on the "thing-a-ma-gig." He called them by their real names, of course, but I never remembered them. I knew what he thought. How did he get a kid who makes straight A's in school but can't remember what a "thing-a-ma-gig" is?

During the winter of my junior year of high school, Dad began his yearly ritual of dismantling the combine. By this time Artie had sold his own combine, and Dad had started cutting Artie's wheat in addition to our own.

Dad parked the combine near the door of the shop. Every Saturday we went out in the cold and started taking off nuts and pulling pins, washing them all with gasoline.

Finally, the guts of the machine were laid out before us; we'd discarded the worn parts and put new ones in their place. It was time to reverse the process and put the combine back together. Dad handed me a sprocket. I had no idea where it went. He took it back and examined it. "On the shaft just inside the wheel," he said.

I tried it. It didn't fit. He tried it. He looked around for another shaft; no luck. Then he handed the sprocket back to me. His eyes were very wide open, his eyebrows high on his forehead. "Keep trying until you find where it goes," he said.

Eventually, I found a shaft the sprocket fit. But what if it wasn't the right sprocket for that shaft? I didn't know. How do you keep track of these things? Dad had always done it, seemingly without thinking.

By late afternoon, we were stymied. Chains and belts were the wrong lengths because sprockets and belt wheels were on the wrong shafts. Dad picked up a crescent wrench and hurled it, denting the cold tin that enclosed the shop. Then he unleashed his rage on me. Why hadn't I been paying attention? Why did I have to think about sports all the time? Why didn't I concentrate on things that were important?

We'd had confrontations in the past, but he hadn't shouted at me for years, not since he became an elder in the church. But what shocked me most was that he started cursing. Dad didn't drink, didn't smoke, and didn't cuss. The only other time I had heard him curse was before he dehorned the registered Herefords.

One of my dad's brothers came over and helped him reassemble the combine. Dad was humiliated.

In the spring of 1957, soon after the confrontation in the shop, my high school sweetheart and I started talking about marriage. Late that summer, we told our parents our plans. We wanted to get married the following summer, after my graduation, and then attend Bible college in South Dakota. My fiancee's dad said she had to be eighteen and graduate from high school before she could get married. She was a year behind me in school, but she took enough courses by correspondence to graduate a year ahead of her class.

Since her eighteenth birthday fell on a Saturday in late July, after harvest, we decided to have the wedding that day. Marrying on the day she turned eighteen symbolized our determination. But there was more to it than that. I also wanted to get away as soon as possible from whatever was happening to my dad.

A few weeks before the wedding, Dad and I cut our wheat and then Artie's wheat. Then we headed north for a couple of weeks, cutting wherever we could find work. When we finished, we trailed the combine home behind the truck, took hot showers, and slept. The next day, we went to Artie's to collect the final payment of the summer. Artie wasn't his usual joking, teasing self. He was sullen and hostile.

"Get in your truck and follow me," Artie told my dad. "I'm gonna show you something fucking goddamned disgusting." I rode silently beside Dad. We arrived at one of the fields we had cut.

"Look at that," Artie said. "I didn't plow it so you could see the shitty job you did." I was looking, but I didn't see anything except a field of wheat stubble. But Dad knew what he was talking about. "Yes, there are a few stalks standing here and there. We'll take something off the bill," he said. Then I saw the wisps of wheat stalks—not many, maybe half a peck of grain per acre left in the field. But the field wasn't clean. Dad always cut clean. It was a matter of pride.

"You'll never see a dime from me for this job," Artie fumed. He flung himself in his truck and drove off, leaving us standing in his field. I felt horrible for Dad. I knew there was no hope of getting the money Artie owed him. Dad and Artie never worked together again.

When we got home, I looked closely at our stubble. It looked the same, maybe even worse.

I didn't know what was wrong with Dad, but I knew something had changed. He couldn't put the combine back together; nor could he drive it as well as he used to.

*

The church was packed the day we got married. Early that evening, we left town for a trip to the Rockies, tin cans dragging behind our car.

A few weeks later, it was time for us to leave for school. Our families milled around the car as we prepared to leave. I shook hands with my dad. His hand was large and rough, his face frozen in a half smile. I shook hands with my father-in-law and pecked my mother-in-law's cheek. My mother was taking motion pictures with a Bell and Howell camera. When I approached her to hug her good-bye, she waved me off, as if filming was more important. I knew she disapproved of my decision to marry at eighteen and to attend Bible college instead of a secular university.

I turned for another look at my dad. He had a blank look on his face, the look I had seen years before on my grandfather, then on my Aunt Pearl. The stress and sadness of the occasion must have triggered it. With the thousand mile stare burned into my mind, my young wife and I got in our car and pulled away.

I looked in the rearview mirror at the buildings lining the wide main street, the grain elevator, and the livestock sale barn where we sold the wild New Mexico cattle. I exhaled a long, slow breath, feeling as if I had escaped some unidentified danger lurking in the sun-baked town.

Chapter Five

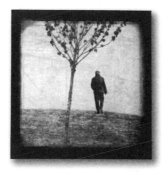

MOVING ON

T *he newest technology of his day enabled Alois Alzheimer to view brain cells in 1906, and observe, draw, and describe the plaques and tangles that have become the identifying characteristics of Alzheimer's disease. When the research on our family began, the technology to observe the plaques and tangles had advanced immeasurably, but still little was known about the plaques (often described to be like wads of gum) and tangles (like matted hair). It was known that both were made of proteins, but no one had been able to crack them open and get inside to see their exact composition. The plaques and tangles were considered to be medical curiosities.*

Dr. George Glenner was well known for his research when he worked for the National Institute of Health in molecular pathology, but, perhaps, is better known as the doctor who helped explain Alzheimer's disease to President and Mrs. Reagan at the White House when the president developed symptoms of the disease.

Dr. Glenner and other colleagues began to study the molecular composition of the plaques and tangles of Alzheimer's in the 1960's. In 1980, Dr. Glenner moved from the NIH to the University of California at San Diego. Then, in 1983, Dr. Glenner unlocked the molecular structure of beta amyloid, the main component of plaques, and, with this discovery, struck the first major blow in the war on Alzheimer's. However, one victory seldom wins a war, and this one precipitated many skirmishes between factions of researchers who were in the same army, all striving to whip Alzheimer's. These battles continue today, largely undecided, and have been termed the fight between the Baptists (scientists who believe beta amyloid protein—plaques—is the culprit in Alzheimer's) and the Tauists (those who believe tau—tangles—is the cause). Have these disagreements between researchers helped or hindered the war on Alzheimer's? The answer may never be known.

🌿

One of the first lessons my wife and I learned after enrolling at the Dakota Bible College had nothing to do with the Bible, theology, or evangelism, but much to with where to buy a trailer house. Using the harvest money I'd earned before our wedding, I'd purchased ours in Amarillo, Texas, but it was built in Georgia. Then we moved it to Huron, South Dakota, and parked it on campus, just across the fence from the Huron airport. Wind blew from the north with nothing to stop it, and it penetrated the walls of our house. When the below-zero air off the northern plains met the just-above-freezing inside our house, it condensed, froze, and formed ice. When we got up in the morning, we chipped ice from the light switch so we could turn on lights, chipped ice from an outlet so we could make coffee, and chipped ice from the door so we could get out and go to class.

I decided to talk to a local trailer house dealer about our problem. The owner wore striped denim overalls like the ones Dad wore when he went to town. I thought this was a good omen. Surely this man could help me. I described the problem, told him we were having a baby in a few months, and asked him how to prevent ice from forming inside the trailer house. He looked me over carefully, then said, "To prevent that from happening, you have to buy a trailer house in the same region of the country where you intend to park it." We bought a space heater.

Every semester I enrolled for twenty credit hours or more and went to summer school so I could graduate in three years. In addition, I worked at a gas station and a meat-packing plant, and I preached at a circuit of rural churches—three or sometimes four sermons per Sunday. On top of all this, our two sons were born during those three years. Thankfully, my parents were helping us get by.

A year after dehorning the registered Herefords, Dad had sold all the beef cows, added a dairy barn, and bought dairy cows. He did this against my mother's wishes as well as mine. (I didn't feel I had any say, though, since I wasn't going to stay on the farm.) Dad said if I used the money from the sale of my registered (dehorned) Herefords to buy dairy cows, he would send me the money from my cows' production while I was in school. This turned out to be a good plan for my family. The supplemental income helped us live reasonably comfortable. But despite the fact that my parents were sending money every month, I gave them little thought.

Since I was preaching regularly and even holding some revival meetings, the president of the Bible college and my hometown minister both thought I should receive the official commission of the church to "preach the gospel." The ordination was scheduled for a Sunday morning as part of the regular church service in my home church. My wife and I loaded up the two babies and drove home.

Dad had been an elder for seven or eight years, and my Uncle George was not only an elder but also a lay preacher. The minister thought it would be fitting for them to offer the ordination prayers.

Mother was worried about Dad participating in the ordination ceremony. She knew he'd feel performance pressure. He'd had some trouble praying in public, especially on occasions such as Easter, when the crowd was unusually large and the congregation's leaders wanted everything to be perfect so the backsliders who came only on Easter Sunday would have nothing to ridicule and might be inspired to become more devoted to the Lord and his church. Sometimes Dad reached a point in his prayer when he could not find the word he wanted, and then he could find no word at all, as if the holy spirit had stopped his tongue. There was a long silence, like those in Quaker meetings, and the congregation shuffled their feet waiting for the "amen" so they could sit down.

For my ordination, Mother helped him write out a short prayer that he memorized. As she drove them to the service, he went over and over the prayer. She told him to keep the prayer in his suit pocket and pull it out just before it was time to pray, in case he needed to read it.

After the sermon, I knelt in front of the baptistery, beneath the picture of the Last Supper, to begin the ordination service. Ordinations usually include a passage from the Apostle Paul's first letter to his young disciple, Timothy. *Do not let people disregard you because you are young, but be an example to all the believers in the way you speak and behave, and in your life, your faith and your purity. Make use of the time until I arrive by reading to the people, preaching, and teaching. You have in you a spiritual gift which was given to you when the prophets spoke and the body of elders laid their hands on you.*[1]

Dad and Uncle George put their hands on my head as I knelt in submission to the will of the Lord. Then the minister called on Dad to offer the first prayer. Silence. Not only had he forgotten the words of the prayer, but he'd also forgotten to take the paper out of his pocket so he could read it.

I could hear the congregation moving restlessly in their seats. I said in a loud whisper, my head still bowed, "Dad, in your pocket."

---

[1] *I Timothy, 4:12-14, The Jerusalem Bible*, Doubleday & Company, Inc. (Garden City 1966).

His left hand was on my head. His right hand searched for the prayer paper, pants pocket, jacket pocket. Then he lifted his hand off my head and checked the other side. He couldn't find it.

The preacher, standing a little behind us, leaned forward and said to my uncle, "Let's go to the next prayer."

Uncle George had been a tail gunner in a bomber during World War II. He had been in some tight situations, but this one befuddled him. He cleared his throat. "Dear Lord," he began. Nothing else came out. He started again, "Dear Lord. . . ."

Like my mother, Aunt Ester May had been worried about whether her husband would forget his prayer for the service. She, too, had helped him prepare. But the task was too much for both Uncle George and Dad.

Finally, mercifully, the preacher stepped forward and prayed a long ordination prayer. I was officially commissioned to "go unto all the world and preach the gospel."

After the service, Mother reached in Dad's suit pocket and found the prayer where he'd put it. Trying to alleviate his embarrassment, she told him, "That kind of thing might happen to anyone. Things turned out fine, so forget it." I turned away, embarrassed as much for Mother as for Dad. What an odd thing to say to him — "forget it." He was already too adept at forgetting.

A month before I graduated from Bible college, an energetic, growing church in Fortville, Indiana, invited me to become their first youth minister. I wanted to accept the job because I had already enrolled for the fall term at Lincoln Christian Seminary, in Lincoln, Illinois, to begin graduate work. I had prayed that the Lord would lead me to a job that would allow me to continue my studies.

Telephone service had finally reached our farm two years after I left home. I called my parents and asked Dad to help me move my family and possessions to Indiana. He agreed to do it, but Mother objected. She didn't want to stay on the farm alone, she claimed. Later she told me her real concern: she didn't want Dad driving long distances by himself. I told her it was an easy drive to South Dakota. After that, he could follow me to Indiana. For the trip home, I'd lay out a course for him to follow.

I was extremely grateful that Dad had agreed to help us. It felt as if he was doing much more than moving our chattel to Indiana. He was helping me launch my life. I vowed I would do the same for my boys when it was time.

Dad drove the 700 miles to South Dakota with no difficulty. After we loaded the truck, I pointed our car toward Indiana and we set out. My dad followed us in the truck, with our belongings protected by grain tarps. We passed through eastern South Dakota, Iowa, and Illinois, past Indianapolis, and into central Indiana. The church elders were there to greet us. They had furnished a house for us.

The next morning, after I marked the easiest route on a map, Dad started back to Oklahoma. Five days later, he had not made it home. He hadn't called Mother to tell her why he was taking so long. I felt terribly guilty about going against her wishes and asking him to drive. I told Mother to call the state police in Oklahoma. I did the same thing in Indiana.

A few hours later, the Oklahoma police called me, and I outlined the route I had suggested to Dad. They found him in Arkansas, well south of the route home. The police in Arkansas put him on the phone with Mother. She asked him, "Why didn't you call me?"

"We don't have a phone," he replied.

"Yes, we do. We put it in two years ago. Remember? You talked to your son on it when you promised him you'd help him move."

She got him to write down the number. He called her every few hours. He made it home two days later.

Chapter Six

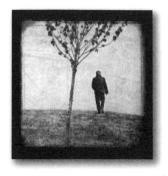

THE PALE HORSE

T *he search for the genes that*
cause early onset Alzheimer's began in the early 1980s, even before
the Alzheimer's Disease Research Centers were funded by the
NIH. The big breakthrough came in 1991 when an early onset
gene and its specific location on chromosome 21 was identified.
The gene was named APP (short for amyloid precursor protein).
Normally, APP protects brain cells. The mutation on APP, how-
ever, interrupts the normal function of the gene causing the help-
ful protein to clump and form the plaques of Alzheimer's. When
the announcement was made of APP's discovery, many thought
this was the familial early onset Alzheimer's gene, but my family
and many others were disappointed to learn that this mutation
was not present in our DNA and the mutation on APP only
accounted for a small percentage of early onset cases.

All brains diseased with Alzheimer's, including those affected
by the malfunctioning APP gene, contain clumps of sticky beta

amyloid protein (BAP). These clumps were what Dr. Alzheimer
observed and called plaques. It appears that the transmission of
messages in the brain is interrupted by the presence of these
plaques because they take up space formerly occupied by transmit-
ters. It was logical to jump to the conclusion that these plaques
cause the disease. However, brains with a significant number of
plaques have been studied post-mortem, yet the individuals had
evidenced no symptoms of Alzheimer's disease before death.

Despite this conundrum, many researchers, termed Baptists
by other researchers, have placed their bets that BAP is the sole or
primary cause of Alzheimer's disease, both early and late onset. To
this date, much of the research money has focused on ways to inter-
rupt the abnormal production of BAP, or, in some cases, to dissolve
and remove the harmful proteins from the brain even after they've
formed. The most well-known of the so-called Baptists is Rudolph
Tanzi, a researcher from Boston prominently involved in the search
for early onset genes.

🍃

W hen we left Dad in the hospital shortly before his death, Mother
drove. The plains were soft green in the early evening light, with
spatters of butter-cups and black-eyed susans on the southern slopes. When
we turned off the highway, onto the road leading to the farm, I rolled down
my window. On the right was the east pasture; I saw the patch of wheat land
I'd been plowing when I got caught in the hail and lighting nearly a decade
ago, the day I gave up my dream of being a baseball player. Since then, I'd
had three children and earned four college degrees, and I was working
toward a Ph.D. As we drove up the road that cut through the farm, the tangy
smell of new sage brush and the dank odor of freshly plowed land were so
familiar I felt as if I'd never been away.

After supper, Mother brought out a small wooden jewelry box. She lifted the lid, reached in, and took out my father's pocketknife. "This should be yours," she said. "I had to take it away from him. He kept cutting himself."

"On purpose?"

"No. But he didn't seem to feel it or think it wasn't normal. He got blood all over the house."

The knife Mother held out to me was less than three inches long, with an ivory handle and two blades, the same knife my father had when I was a boy. I lost my pocket knives all the time. Yet, despite all the memory and organizational problems he'd had, Dad had never lost his.

I hesitated to take the knife. What if Dad needed it? By offering it to me, Mother was declaring that Dad's life was over. She placed it on the table and slid it across to me. "I know he'd want you to have it, after all the things you two did together."

In bed, at the edge of sleep, I listened to an alternating chorus of crickets near the house and frogs in the creek. It seemed as if they were singing to each other—a cross-species, discordant concert. I thought of Dad in the hospital, the way he floated in and out of reality, sometimes present and almost himself, and sometimes on another planet. He might never hear this cacophony of country music again.

*

There was a knock on my door. "Get up," Dad said, "I need your help."

I'd already gotten up earlier, I was ten, not yet into the heavy morning sleep of adolescence, to let a tabby kitten climb through the window into my room. Every morning she mewed until I let her in and petted her. I pulled on my clothes, and joined Dad at the breakfast table. Mother, without speaking or looking at me, slammed a plate of ham, eggs, and toast across the battered wood. She glanced at Dad, menace in her eyes. He ate silently, looking at his plate.

"What are we doing today?" I asked.

"The calves need to be worked," Dad said.

I hoped he didn't mean "dehorned." That was the work I hated most, the bloodiest and the most painful for the calves. I wasn't like the men I worked with; unlike me, they all seemed immune to the pain we caused our animals.

It turned out the calves needed to be vaccinated, and the bulls had to be castrated, except those registered to sell as breeders. Castration may be as painful as dehorning, but at least there's much less bleeding.

We saddled the two bay horses, Dusty and Lady. We crossed the road into the east pasture and headed southeast in a canter. Dad rode slightly ahead of me. He and Lady seemed like one form, flowing together in a gentle up and down. I bounced along on Dusty, a horse-length behind them, the saddle rising when I fell, slapping my butt.

Hearing this, Dad asked, "Can you get in rhythm with him?"

"He has no rhythm," I said.

We saw the cows and calves on the hillside in the far southeast corner of the pasture, nearly a mile away. Dad stopped, cupped his hands around his mouth, and called a high, piercing "Aaahweeeeoooooooo!" The cows recognized this call, picked up their heads, and looked. Deep in the winter, when the grass was no longer so lush, they'd come running when they heard this call because they knew it meant there was hay to eat. But today they had plenty to eat and saw no truck loaded with hay, only two riders on horseback—which only meant trouble.

"They're not cooperating," Dad said. "Gonna make us ride all the way out there to bring them in."

We reached the cattle and started moving them toward the house. Some of the cows bawled for their calves in the tones of mothers searching for lost children. Most of the calves trotted alongside their mothers, but some of the older ones were frisky and darted around.

Dad rode Lady with one hand holding the reins and the other on his hip. She was a smart filly. Dad barely touched the reins when they went after a wayward calf. I had to use all my strength to turn Dusty—jug-headed, hard-mouthed Dusty—but within a few minutes, all the cows and calves were paired up and headed in the same direction. They intersected the trail and walked single file toward the barn. They seemed to know they had no choice in the matter and might as well get it over with.

An hour later, we had all fifty head of cows and calves in the large holding pen.

Dad caught a stout young bull. I held him down, and Dad vaccinated him. Then he took a small whetstone out of his pocket and sharpened his knife.

"Watch exactly what I do," he said. I had helped him do this a hundred times, it seemed, but I didn't like to watch when he opened the calf's scrotum to cut out the testicles. I usually closed my eyes. This time, I kept them open and watched.

He punctured the scrotum with the point of his knife. The calf flinched, bellowed, and flailed his head, banging it on the ground. Dad put one foot on the calf's neck to keep him from hurting himself. "You make a wide cut at the bottom of the bag so it will drain and not get infected," he said. "Then you can reach in, like this." He took hold of the testicles with his left hand and then slid the scrotum up with the other hand, the same hand that held his knife. He cut the two white veiny looking roots where they got thin, smoothed the scrotum back, checked the opening again to make sure it was large enough, then painted the whole scrotum, now nothing more than a wrinkled sack of skin, with a brush dipped in disinfectant.

I kept hold of the rope, but turned the calf's legs loose. The calf stood up. His legs shook. We dragged him to the gate. His mother sniffed him, blew out her breath, and made a lowing, throaty sound. We put them out. Dad handed me the rope.

"This time, I'll be your helper," he said. I realized he'd given this moment some thought. That's what he and Mother had been arguing about at breakfast. She thought I was too young to be castrating animals.

I lengthened the loop on the lasso and caught a calf. It was a heifer. I glanced at Dad. He avoided looking at me; I knew he knew I'd caught a heifer on purpose. We threw her down on her side. Dad held her, and I got the vaccination gun.

"What did you do wrong?" he asked me.

"I didn't get the vaccine prepared first," I said. While he kept the calf down, I inserted the needle in the rubber top of the vaccine bottle, carefully extracted the vaccine by pulling out the plunger, and shot her in the hip without mishap.

"Well done," Dad said. He let her up, and we took her and her mother outside the corral.

I prepared the vaccine and caught another calf. This time I caught a bull, because I knew I couldn't delay any longer. We put him down on the ground. I expected Dad to hand me his knife. Instead, he gave me a new knife. It had a brown bone handle. "I got this for you," he said. "I've sharpened it because they don't come very sharp from the factory. You'll have to keep it sharp. The pointed blade should be used for castrations. You can cut other stuff with the short blade."

I opened the longer blade, approached the calf, reached between his legs, and made the long cut for drainage. I slid the scrotum up, exposing the testicles, and cut them out exactly the way he showed me. I finished with the disinfectant. Dad let the calf up and said, "Real good. Do one more, and I'll finish up. You'll get faster the more you do it. Well done—very well done." He flicked the bill of my baseball cap. I wiped the knife blade on my pants leg like I'd seen him do, folded the blade into its slot, and dropped it in my pocket. I prepared the vaccine and then took the rope and caught another calf, making sure I got a bull.

On Monday, I took my new knife to school and showed it around. None of the other boys had ever castrated a calf. Just before school ended, I reached into my pocket. No knife! I panicked. What would my dad say? I told the teacher I'd lost it. She let me go outside to look around. I stumbled around the area where I'd been showing my knife to the other boys. I was still looking when school let out. Mother walked across the schoolyard toward me. I kept my head down, looking intently.

"Mrs. Nicholson told me what happened," she said. "I'll help you look." We kept searching for ten or fifteen minutes.

Finally, Mother said, "We have to get home to help your dad with the chores. Maybe you'll find it tomorrow." Tears leaked out and rolled down my cheeks. "If you're worried about your dad, I'll tell him what happened," Mother said. I nodded.

On the way home, I remembered a small white-handled knife Artie Evans gave me when I was three. It was hardly an inch long, with one tiny blade. It served no practical purpose, but it was mine. Soon enough I lost it, and soon after that we moved. Mother sometimes let me walk the mile back to our old property to look for it.

As we drove home from school, I said, "Remember the knife Artie gave me? I never found it, and I probably won't find this one. Why did I have to lose it?" I sobbed uncontrollably. That didn't feel right for a boy my age.

***

It was light when I woke up. I looked at the window to see if the kitten was on the sill. Then I realized I wasn't in my old room anymore, or my old house. Dad wouldn't call me to come help him bring in the cattle. This was the new house Uncle Otto had built for Mom and Dad. Dad would never call me again for anything.

***

After Dad's burial, we left the cemetery in the funeral car. As the mortician picked up speed on the open road, I tried to control my emotions. On the left, in a northwesterly direction, I could see town, the elevator, the sale barn, a line of tamaracks and cottonwoods along the river. On the right, the open prairie stretched southeasterly past the farm of my Uncle George and Aunt Ester May, toward our farm, twenty miles away.

I could see things clearly now. We had expected my father's death, and—God forgive us if it was wrong—had even wished for it and prayed for it. But now that he was gone, I suddenly saw myself standing next in line. I was still in my mid-twenties, nowhere near ready to be a family patriarch. But here I was, the oldest male in a line of men who died young.

Because of his diminished capacity to provide leadership and guidance, in some ways my father had been dead to us for a long time. And yet his death was so terribly slow. Grandmother's sudden, violent death at the Huntoon crossing made more sense than the elongated draining of mental capacity my grandfather and my father had suffered.

As the funeral car turned onto the highway heading back to the church, I pulled my three-year-old daughter onto my lap and held her. But there was little comfort for me in looking to the next generation. If I had inherited the gene from my father as my father had from his, then my children could also get it from me. I wanted to protect them from illness, but I couldn't. They had my genes. All I could do was protect them from the fear, and that meant protecting them from knowledge. But that wouldn't be fair or right.

What little we knew, and what we were learning, about our family problem must be brought into the family dialogue and acknowledged. The secrecy must end. Although I vowed to do my part to end it, fear raked me. Still, I knew I must stay calm and focused on my career, family, and calling. I had to resist the desire to buck off the unwelcome weight of responsibility I acquired upon my father's death.

Chapter Seven

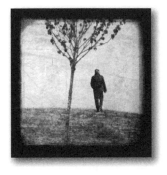

HOW MUCH TIME
IS ENOUGH?

The *tangles described by Dr. Alzheimer in 1906 contain a different protein from that identified in the plaques. The protein in the tangles is named tau. A minority of researchers working to cure Alzheimer's believe that tau plays the major role in the disease, and, that the plaques comprised of beta amyloid protein are the result of the disease, not the cause, much like scar tissue is the result of an injury. The researchers who believe the failure of tau is the major cause of Alzheimer's have been termed Tauists.*

The brain contains axons that carry the signals from one nerve cell to another. The protein tau supports these axons like railroad ties support tracks enabling freight to move smoothly and safely through the country. When tau deteriorates into tangles, the axons die and the signals that the brain sends to control our every thought and action are interrupted, or wrecked. Mutations in the tau genes have been found to cause diseases similar to Alzheimer's where there are tangles present but few or no plaques, lending credence to the views of the Tauists.

When I was three, Dad sat me on his lap and taught me how to steer the truck. When I was five, he put me on my knees on the truck seat and told me steer while he jumped on the back of the truck to feed hay. It was one thing to guide the truck while I was on Dad's lap with his muscular arms around me; it was another to steer while I was alone in the truck's cab, the gears grinding, the truck rocking from side to side over the prairie terrain. To allay my fears when he disappeared onto the back, Dad pointed to a landmark far in the distance and said, "Keep your eyes on where you're going."

After my father died, my own passage through death's door seemed imminent, as if he'd left it open for me. I calculated I had more than ten years before my mind would begin to short-circuit from the plaques and tangles of Alzheimer's. But looking back at how quickly the past ten years had sped by, it seemed as if the next decade could end tomorrow.

Thoughts careened through my head. I made mental notes to myself. Take vitamins. Look into macrobiotic diets. Remember, knowledge is the only thing of value. But contradictory thoughts came in the other side of my brain. Education is a waste. You'll forget everything. Live more.

From the time I was baptized at age nine, I'd been taught to seek answers in prayer. But now, no matter how much I prayed, I didn't feel better, or more hopeful. I wasn't so depressed that my life went off track. I did my job. I preached. I baptized. I visited the sick and prayed with them. I conducted funerals. Nor do I think my family noticed much change in me after Dad's death. We went to the amusement park, to Pirates' games, on picnics. But everything I did felt empty. My sense of purpose had evaporated. When Dad died, my core seemed to melt.

I had always felt that living near the poverty line helped maintain my devotion to Christ and to the ministry. But after Dad died, I thought about how hard he had worked and how few of life's amenities he'd enjoyed. I started to think that being poor was antithetical to a satisfying life. I didn't need to be rich — just a little bit more comfortable. I thought a Ph.D. might help, so I concentrated on my studies. Study more, live more became my motto.

I heard footsteps on the stairs. It was my one o'clock counseling appointment. I was hoping to finish my sermon so I could take Saturday off and be with my family. I glanced at the door to make sure it was open, and then I kept typing.

When I swiveled my chair away from the typewriter, one of my congregrants was standing in the doorway. She wore a floral sundress and sandals. Her blonde, wavy hair was cut in a pageboy and brushed to a sheen. She was smiling, showing her strong white teeth. I stood up, welcomed her, guided her to the chair in front of my desk, closed the door, and, as usual, sat behind the desk. A cloud crossed her face.

She glanced around the room and noticed another side chair. Her voice was soft, with a slight waver, as if she needed to clear her throat. "Could you sit in this other chair?" she asked.

I feel a pang of guilt at having put the heavy wooden desk between us. Perhaps I was trying to convey how busy I was. I pulled up the chair and leaning toward her, I chided myself: "Give her your full attention, no matter how long it takes. She needs your help or she wouldn't be here. The sermon can wait."

She folded her dress under her legs so the fabric was stretched tight against her thighs, and left her fingers tucked under them as if for warmth. She wore no makeup. Her lips, pink and full, needed no adornment. Her eyes were pale blue, with dark lashes. Other than a few freckles, her skin was very white, as if she'd avoided all contact with the sun. I waited for her to speak.

"I've never done anything like this before," she said.

I could barely hear her, "What do you mean by 'anything like this'?"

Her head drooped forward. Her lashes fluttered, then closed. I thought she might faint. Without looking up, she spoke again—so quietly I wasn't sure I heard her, and yet I knew I hadn't missed a single syllable. "I've never made an appointment with a man to ask him to sleep with me."

I absorbed what she'd said and waited for her to continue. When she spoke again, her voice was stronger. Her words flowed out in torrents. "There's no turning back now," she said. "I'm prepared to have you say whatever you have to say. Tell me to go to hell, which is probably where you think I'm going. Tell me I'm a whore. That would be a relief, to have someone I truly respect tell me that. I know you see inside me. When you preach, you know what I'm thinking. I'm not telling you anything you don't already know. You already know I feel this way. You know you can do whatever you want to me. Even if you kick me out, slap me, I'll feel thankful, and blessed, as long as you're honest and tell me what you think and feel. I can't take any more dishonesty. I want someone to tell me the truth."

I remained very still.

"I don't think I'm horrible for thinking about this," she said. "It's consuming me, but it's fulfilling me at the same time. It's the only thing that means anything right now." She paused, and her voice softened again. "Tell me the truth. Have you ever thought of doing anything like that with anyone besides your wife?"

Her question relieved my tension. I could answer her question, tell her the truth. What was the harm in that? Isn't truth the core of redemption and forgiveness? I pushed aside the thought that, perhaps, my own floodgates might open, and that, perhaps, I shouldn't answer. I admitted to her that I had, recently, begun to wonder what it would be like to make love with another woman.

"Why so recently?" she asked. "I know you've been married ten years. That's a long time for someone under thirty. I've only been married two, and I'm already desperate."

"I think it might have to do with the death of my dad," I told her. "I feel life is so short, and I have done so little living, and I may not have much more time. If I have ten years left to live at full capacity, do you think that will be enough to have lived a life?"

She shrugged. The question did not seem very relevant to her. She didn't know anything about my family or about the gene. So I told her about my grandfather and the accident at the Huntoon crossing, about my dad who couldn't pray at my ordination and who got lost going home from Indiana, and about my uncles and aunts. It seemed she listened as no one had ever listened to me before. Over the months I knew her and met her for afternoons in her sister's apartment, the floodgates opened. I told her I did not know what I believed anymore, did not think prayer changed anything, suffering was random and purposeless. The core was missing. I had to focus my eyes on a new destination.

When the relationship ended, my marriage fell apart, and my family moved back to the small town in Oklahoma where my wife and I both came from. By then I believed that what we get in life is all there is, and for me, that included a fifty-fifty chance of having Alzheimer's within the next decade or two.

With the Ph.D. in hand, I began looking toward the horizon, finding what was now important so I could steer toward it.

Chapter Eight

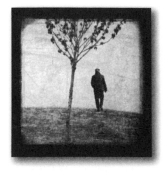

MY HANDSOME UNCLE
AND BEAUTIFUL AUNT

S*everal major pharmaceutical
companies have entered the race to find treatments and cures for
Alzheimer's disease. These companies have spent millions, now
turning to billions, for research and testing. The four or five drugs
currently available to treat the disease have shown mixed results.
But that does not stop people from using them and spending
money on them because Alzheimer's creates a state of desperation
among people with the disease and those who care for them. So
families make financial sacrifices on the chance that one drug, or
a combination of several, may help slow down the deterioration of
the brain. It is this market the pharmaceutical companies are
competing for.*

*At last count, the NIH supports twenty-two studies that are
trying to find treatments for Alzheimer's. Other studies are financed*

privately. Many of these studies aim to stop the process wherein the beta amyloid proteins clump together and form the plaques that some researchers assume are the major cause of Alzheimer's. However, recently more grants have been given to people studying tau. It appears inevitable that there will be treatments for abnormalities in both plaques and tangles. There is a further minority opinion that neither beta amyloid nor tau holds the key to treatment of the disease. When the new generation of drugs come on the market, these continuing scientific debates make it seem unlikely one drug will be the cure-all for everyone, and, possibly, one drug alone will not be a totally effective treatment for anyone.

When I was six, what I wanted most for Christmas was a metal truck I'd seen in the Montgomery Ward catalog. But metal toys were expensive, so instead of the truck, I got a coping saw. It came with several extra blades of different widths. The narrower the blade, the easier it was to turn while sawing. But the narrow blades broke easily.

My dad said, "With this saw, you can make your own truck." Of course, since I was only six, I'd need his help. And he was busy. We made something easier—a rifle, sawed from pine. Dad showed me how to put my knee on the board to hold it steady while I sawed. He bent over me, placed my hand on the saw handle, put his hand over my hand, and guided the motion. Soon I could do it myself. I cut most of the straight lines, and he sawed most of the curves and drilled the hole for my trigger finger. He let me use the silver reflective paint he used on the water tank, so the gun looked like metal.

On the day my uncle Otto was expected to come home from the war, I climbed up the water tank with my gun, and I plopped down on my stomach so I could watch the road. I had the gun nestled in the crook of my arm while I looked toward the highway. That's the direction my uncle would be coming from.

It didn't bother me that I was twenty feet off the ground, on a flat tank with no railing. My mother didn't like me to go up there, but until she forbade it, I spent a lot of time on top of the tank, playing. It was a matter of perspective. I felt intelligent and alert there, above it all.

The sun was hot on my bare back. I was getting thirsty and thought I might have to climb down for a drink. There was a faucet inside the well house, but I wondered if I could I get a drink from the tank. There was a lid on top, large enough for a man to fit through for cleaning, right at my feet. I put my gun aside and grabbed the lid. It wouldn't budge. I sat up and kicked one end and the lid turned, an inch or two, then half a turn, and then I could turn it with my arms. I got it loose, but I needed to stand up to lift the heavy lid out of its opening. When I stood up, I saw my uncle. He was already halfway down the hill. He wore his green Army uniform and a hat with a narrow bill, and he carried a duffle bag over his shoulder. He had hitchhiked from Fort Chaffee, Arkansas, where he'd received his discharge papers.

I forgot my thirst, left the lid half off the opening, and flattened myself on the tank. As long as I lay still, I didn't think he'd see me.

I knew Dad hadn't gone to the war because he was a farmer, and farmers were needed to stay home and grow food and pay taxes. But Uncle Otto had been a farmer, too. After the Huntoon crossing accident, Granddad could no longer do the farming. When Uncle Otto recovered from the accident and graduated from high school, he managed the 640-acre farm. He kept doing so until he was drafted, in the summer of 1942. The local draft board didn't make him report for duty until after harvest.

After Uncle Otto's call-up, Mother was afraid that Dad would be called, too. But Uncle Otto was eight years younger than Dad, and unmarried. That made a big difference. Dad never got his notice from the draft board to report for active duty.

I was glad Dad was home and safe; I knew some men with children had enlisted and had been killed, and I didn't want Dad to die except when he spanked me. But I wasn't entirely satisfied with the farmer excuse, either. I admired my uncles who had gone to the war, especially Otto, the one who had survived the wreck that killed my grandmother, and the last of my uncles to come home from the war. After he trained in Wisconsin, he served for nearly three years in Europe, driving trucks in the medical service, continuing our family's support of the Seventh Day Adventist philosophy of pacifism.

Uncle Otto was the handsomest member of our family. I wasn't the only one who thought so. I had heard my mother and her younger sister, Betty, talking about him. Betty wasn't married yet, and she was at least as interested in Otto's homecoming as I was. She would be disappointed she had not been at our house when he arrived.

As I watched Uncle Otto from on top of the water tank, I examined his swagger. When my dad walked, his feet turned slightly outward, but my uncle walked like an Indian, toe to heel, feet pointed straight ahead. I wondered if they taught him that in the Army. I felt a fullness welling up in my throat; I was intensely proud to be related to this handsome man in a uniform. I wanted to know everything about him. Above all, I wanted to be as tall as he was. But first I wanted to try on his hat.

I squelched my excitement as he approached the well house. After he passed beneath me, I stood up, pointed my gun at the middle of his back, and shouted as loudly as I could, "Hands up!" He jumped and spun around.

"You little scamp," he said. "You scared me. Look how you've grown. Get down from there before you fall."

"I won't fall," I said.

"But come down so I can see you," he said. "I'm not coming up there. It's too high for me."

The ribbons pinned to his jacket scratched my cheek when he hugged me against his chest. His clothing smelled like a sweaty animal. I broke away and ran ahead to tell my mother and sister he was here, then dashed back so I could be with him when they came outside. My sister came first. Although she was nine and gangly, he lifted her higher than his head. Then he set her down and opened his arms for my mother, whose head fit neatly under his chin. Her mane of blonde hair stood out against his uniform as they embraced. I started to get impatient. I wanted to show him my gun, but I'd left it in the house when I ran in to spread the news.

We all went inside. Mother knew Otto must be tired after hitchhiking all the way from Arkansas. She told him to get some sleep. She also said she'd invite his brothers and sisters for supper. My sister and I were ecstatic. Our uncle was home from the war! He was staying with us and would sleep in our room while we slept in the living room. We couldn't wait to tell our cousins.

After Otto woke up from his nap, I showed him my gun. He asked me if I had made it myself, and I said I had; I didn't tell him Dad had helped me. While I was showing him I could twirl it on my finger, Dad came home. He and Uncle Otto shook hands. Although Otto was considerably taller, I saw how much they looked alike, and it made me feel warm and close to Dad.

"So what do you think of this guy? He's grown, hasn't he?" Dad asked Otto, nodding his head toward me. "He's been drinking his milk," he added.

"He ambushed me from on top of the water tank," my uncle said. "I thought I'd been shot in the back."

I asked Uncle Otto, "Did you shoot anybody in the war?" He and Dad both laughed.

"You don't need to know that," my uncle said.

Uncle Otto didn't marry my mother's younger sister, Betty. He married a tall, beautiful, eighteen-year-old girl named Marie, from west of town. Marie had a beehive stack of shiny black hair and wore eye makeup, lipstick, and store-bought dresses instead of the homemade dresses my mother and Betty wore. My cousins and I thought our new aunt was the most beautiful woman we had ever seen, a perfect wife for our handsome uncle. At family gatherings, we boys teased her. She'd say, "If you don't stop that, I'm going to kiss you." We kept teasing, pretending we were disgusted by her threat. So she'd get out her lipstick and refresh her lips, pretend she was paying no attention, and when we got close enough, she'd grab us and leave her lips' imprint on our cheeks.

Uncle Otto and Aunt Marie had two children, Anne and Karl. Anne had smooth olive skin like her mother, and large dark eyes. Karl was tall and rangy like his dad. Uncle Otto, a skilled mechanic and carpenter, started his own carpentry business, and he built a new house for their family in town.

Aunt Marie was easy to talk to, and, unlike many other members of the family, tolerant of Aunt Ester May's foibles. But like my mother, Aunt Marie objected to how much Aunt Ester May talked about Alzheimer's after the disease was diagnosed in Uncle George and Dad. Ultimately, however, unlike other family members, she supported Ester May's decision to place Uncle George in a veteran's hospital.

Uncle Otto was only three years younger than Uncle George. Pearl, Dad, and George had started showing symptoms of Alzheimer's in their forties or earlier, but Otto seemed fine. Then, in his early fifties, he began to have difficulty keeping track of his business finances. Aunt Marie tried to help him, but he was uncharacteristically impatient and edgy.

Like a child convinced there is something frightening under the bed, we can all have trouble separating imagined fears from reality. In our family, however, we tended to deny the existence of trouble where trouble existed. After Uncle Otto started to show symptoms, Aunt Marie knew she must check under the bed, even though she hoped she was only imagining things.

In 1973, when Otto was fifty-four, Aunt Marie took him to the University of Oklahoma Medical Center. Tests indicated "disturbed visual-spatial and visual-temporal problem solving abilities, mildly impaired memory functioning, and moderately impaired nonverbal information." The findings were "felt to be compatible with a presenile dementia rather than the result of the normal aging process."

Ten years had elapsed since Dad and Uncle George had been to the same facility. In that decade, the medical profession had learned a great deal about our family, and our family had begun to face up to the family problem.

*

Uncle Otto, who had survived the deadly Huntoon crossing accident, soon became a danger to himself and other workers at his carpentry business.

After he stopped working, Aunt Marie got a job so they'd have some money coming in. By then, their children, Anne and Karl, were grown and married. When the grandkids arrived, Uncle Otto held them on his knee. But this stage didn't last long. Soon Uncle Otto couldn't be left home alone; if he decided to cook something, he was liable to burn the house down. Then he became incontinent and belligerent and refused to accept Aunt Marie's help. Finally, she placed him in the veterans' hospital in Clinton, Oklahoma.

When Uncle Otto could no longer eat, the hospital requested permission to insert a feeding tube into his stomach. He'd starve otherwise, they told my beautiful Aunt Marie. What was a wife to do? She'd married a handsome man who had survived the Dust Bowl and a severe accident and came home healthy from the war. She couldn't let him starve, so she gave her permission.

As Uncle Otto shrank from a strapping, raw-boned man, to a one hundred-pound corpse with a still-beating heart, Marie realized the feeding tube was a mistake, and she withdrew her permission. But it was too late. The medical staff refused to remove the feeding tube and told her she'd need a court order. She started the process but found the procedures onerous and overwhelming, and the questions unanswerable. When my uncle's weight dropped to seventy-one pounds, he died. He had lived nearly ten years longer than any of his siblings who had the early onset Alzheimer's gene. The same life force that helped him survive the deadly accident at Huntoon contributed to his own elongated suffering, and that of his family.

Chapter Nine

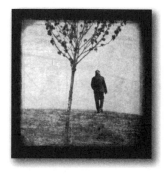

LIVING THE LIFE,
DYING THE DEATH

T*he first scientific article that
included research about our family was published in 1979.*[1] *The
article came out of the Department of Neurology at the University
of Colorado. A circular pedigree chart, adapted from one hand-
drawn by Aunt Ester May, showed those members of our family
who had early onset Alzheimer's disease, represented by either a
black box for men or a black circle for women. When the University of Colorado was unable to continue the research, our family
became involved with Doctors Bird and Schellenberg at the
University of Washington Alzheimer's Disease Research Center.*

---

[1] Robert H. Cook, Brian E. Ward, and James H. Austin. *Studies in aging of the brain:
IV. Familial Alzheimer disease: Relation to transmissible dementia, aneuploidy, and
microtubular defects,* NEUROLOGY, 29: 1402–1412, October 1979.

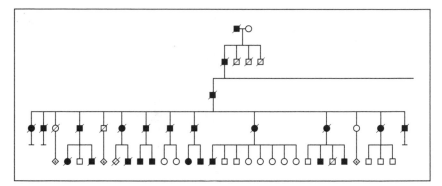

Pedigree of the R family, the largest family with Alzheimer's disease yet reported, showing a pattern of autosomal dominant transmission.

Ultimately, they drew a different form of chart similar to the one I have included above.

In my grandfather's generation, there were two other brothers who had the disease, so there were other affected branches. At the time, our family had more early onset cases than any other family in the United States, and, so far as I know, this is still the case. The chart I am using includes only my granddad's branch, beginning with Jacob and Anna who arrived in the United States in 1878, through my generation, which is still in the process of finding out how many of the twenty-five children of affected parents have inherited the gene. At the moment, the number stands at ten. Even as the count in my generation continues, the oldest of the next generation (not included on the chart) is coming into the age of onset.

The devastation in my father's generation with at least ten of fourteen affected led the early researchers to wonder about the likelihood of an autosomal dominant gene as the cause of the disease and to theorize about viruses and environmental causes. Nevertheless, eventually we learned about the gene and its statistical possibilities. The first black circle represents Aunt Pearl. She married Uncle Bob in her forties and they had no children. As the *oldest, she was the first to become forgetful. One sister described her as "dotty." The next box is my Uncle Oliver. He did not have PS2, the early onset gene, but he did have two copies of ApoE4, the so-called susceptibility gene and had Alzheimer's at age sixty-eight and died at seventy-eight. He and Aunt Thelma had no biological children, but adopted a boy and a girl. The fourth child, a black box, is my dad. He was officially diagnosed at age fifty. The seventh sibling is Uncle George. He "became irritable and impotent at age forty. . . . At forty-five, he could no longer understand how to do even the simplest constructions needed for carpentry. At age fifty, in a vegetative state, he was transferred to a chronic care facility. He had recurrent seizures, frequent myoclonus, and decorticate posturing, and was completely mute".² The ninth sibling was Uncle Otto. Onset was later than the others, fifty-six, and he died at seventy-four, comatose, weighing seventy-one pounds. The eleventh was Aunt Reba (see Chapter 13). She was "disoriented for time, place, and person. She was depressed, and had become apathetic, untidy, and careless. . . . Alzheimer [sic] disease was the sole cause of death noted on her death certificate."³*

In 1979, with our family's age of onset for Alzheimer's disease bearing down on me, my second wife, Rita, our one year-old son, Jesse, and I moved from Pittsburgh to East Hampton, New York, where we had purchased the Maidstone Arms, a venerable hotel on Main Street. Twelve years had elapsed since Dad died. He had only lived two decades after Granddad died. My sister, two and a half years older than I, was becoming forgetful. Mother was worried, not only about her, but about my younger brother and me.

---

² *Ibid.*
³ *Ibid.*

Rita and I knew about the Alzheimer's gene in my family when we married, and we wrestled with the question of whether to have a child. But when Rita's 30th birthday came and went, we stopped using birth control and flipped the genetic coin.

After Jesse was born, we struggled to balance work and family. Rita was the director of a children's therapeutic clinic; I had left the ministry and completed my Ph.D., and I'd become a community planner for the City of Pittsburgh planning department, with special assignments in education and historic preservation.

Sometimes I yearned for a life like my parents had, where labor and the return from the work were tied together inextricably. I yearned to be my own boss. If I began to lose my mind, I wanted to work as long as possible, just as Dad had kept working on the farm with Mother's help. I didn't want to be under a boss who could fire me the moment I slipped up.

I also had dreams of being a writer—a dream that required a lot more free time. With those thoughts in mind, and building on my experience in historic preservation, Rita and I decided to buy the Maidstone. As we imagined it, we'd live in a summer resort community and keep the hotel open for six months a year. I could write my novel in the winter, and, when Jesse was ready for school, Rita could resume her career as a psychotherapist.

And so, in June of 1979, we moved to East Hampton, New York, and became the new owners of the Maidstone Arms. We opened the hotel for the July 4th weekend. In six months I would be forty—just about the age when we began to notice subtle changes in the behavior and mental acuity of my dad, my uncles, and my aunts.

🍂

Our first guest walked in the door. He was a tall, thin young man with a face marked by a bad case of teenage acne. He said he was looking for a waiter's job in the Hamptons and needed a room for one night. He paid us forty dollars for a room with a private bath.

After we closed on the property, the former owner had given us a quick course in hotel management. Since he had owned the inn for more than a decade, we took his advice and adopted his policies. Rule number one: "Collect all room fees in advance and never, never return money for any reason. Otherwise word will get around that you're soft, and people will take advantage of you."

Our first guest had been in his room for about a half hour when he reappeared at the desk and said he'd decided to drive on to Montauk, where he knew some people he could stay with. He wanted his money back. I explained our policy.

After arguing for a while, he said he knew "some people who could take care of this problem." He called the shingled inn a tinderbox. "Now give me my money back," he insisted.

Doubt clouded my mind. Why had I thought I was capable of running a hotel? Perhaps the whole idea was a symptom of Alzheimer's—*poor or decreased judgment*—like Dad's idea to buy the wild cattle from New Mexico.

Still, I refused to reimburse him. He stomped across the wooden porch, shaking his fist. "You have not heard the last of me!" he shouted.

Although we'd collected our first payment, I was shaken by the experience. If our first guest turned out to be this troublesome, things could only get worse. But other guests arrived and were happy.

After we got the rooms open, the next step was to open the restaurant. To do that, we needed a liquor license. We obtained all the forms from the New York State Liquor Control Board, filled them out, and sent them in. Months later, I received a letter asking for more information—information I thought I'd already supplied.

My wife, always watching for the dreaded forgetfulness, asked me what was going on. I said I was sure the board had made a mistake. But beneath my bravado, I thought maybe *I* had made a mistake, the kind people make in the early phases of Alzheimer's disease. I put the information in the envelope and sent it back. Our Liquor Control Board rep replied immediately. He told us we'd have to meet with him in his office. At this point, the application process had already taken eight months.

We drove to Hauppauge for the meeting. Instead of explaining what was missing from our application, the rep rambled on about how long he had been employed by the LCB, how many children he had, how much dentistry cost, and how he hoped to take his kids to Disneyland. He handed us a brown envelope and asked us to send it back, addressed to him personally, with some "additional information," the same information I thought I'd already sent twice. No—now I was *sure* I had. And that in itself—knowing my memory was not to blame—was a huge relief, although it didn't solve our problem.

We met with the attorney who had handled our purchase of the Maidstone Arms, and told him what was going on with the liquor license. He advised us to play it straight. "If they catch you offering a bribe, you'll never get a license."

That week I bumped into the mayor of East Hampton Village, Kenneth Wessberg. He asked how things were going and I and mentioned the problem we were having getting a liquor license. A week later, our license arrived in the mail. Later I found out that the mayor contacted a friend at the LCB; this friend waited until our rep was out to lunch, pulled our application out of the pile on his desk, and walked it through the system.

After we opened the restaurant, I realized that being an innkeeper was far from the perfect profession for someone who was worried about his memory. Sometimes not much at all happened. Other times, ten things happened at once—one guest wanted to check in early, another one checked out late, the phone rang, the wine distributor arrived and wanted his delivery approved pronto so he could get home early, the phone rang again, and the second line rang at the same time.

One morning I took a wine delivery to the basement. When I'd stacked all ten cases at the bottom of the basement stairs, I suddenly remembered a phone message I'd forgotten to give one of our guests, Mrs. Green. Her husband had called and asked me to tell her he'd be an hour late for their meeting in town. I dashed back up to give Mrs. Green her message, but she had already left for the meeting. "Something's wrong," I thought, "I have to learn how to keep things in my head."

A half hour later, the chef stomped into my office. "You forgot to put your wine away. It's stacked at the bottom of the stairs. How do you expect me to get to my supplies?" he yelled.

I devised systems of reminders, including sticky notes and a notebook by the phone to record every call. This reminded me of the ways Mother tried to keep Dad organized.

By the mid 1980s, I had reached the prime age of onset for my family's disease. By then, the Maidstone wine cellar contained an impressive collection of fine wines.

I decided that if I was getting Alzheimer's, I'd use these wines to help me take my own life, sparing my family the prolonged agony of my illness. My plan danced along the edges of farm-boy practicality, wine snobbery, and insanity. But it would keep my children and wife from having to pray for my death, as Mother and I had prayed for my dad to be taken.

I'd wait as long as I could, and then use my last reserves of intellectual capacity to take several bottles of wine to the beach on a near-zero day. I'd keep to the back of the dunes so no one walking along the beach would see me. I'd drink the wines from lightest to heaviest, starting with Chateau Mouton Rothschild, then Jordan or Chateau Montelena from California, and ending with Petrus, a deep purple French wine of great depth and intensity. Although alcohol makes you feel warm when you drink it, it constricts the blood vessels, which increases the speed of hypothermia. After each bottle I downed, I'd take off a layer of clothes. I'd drink until I passed out and let hypothermia do the job. To me, this kind of death had a unique symmetry, since I'd been born in the middle of a blizzard that had nearly killed my father.

I also thought that numbing myself with great wines was a more pleasant way to go than drowning myself or blowing out my brains with a gun. My plan, however, didn't address all of my family's feelings. I'd have to kill myself without preparing them beforehand; they'd feel obligated to stop me if I mentioned my plan. At the very least, I'd have to write a note, a letter, *something* to explain my actions. I had to tell them I loved them, tell them why I believed I was doing something considerate rather than selfish, by sparing them five, ten, or even more years of caring for a man who probably wouldn't even know he was being cared for. Most of all, I'd have to assure them that I had done what I felt was right.

Chapter Ten

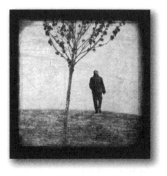

INSIDE OUT

Science has long described the progression of Alzheimer's disease as reverse development. My aunt Ester May confirmed that Uncle George's progression through Alzheimer's was exactly that. First he went from being an adult to an adolescent: moody, sometimes belligerent, overly opinionated, and erratic. Then he progressed backward through all the stages of childhood until he was a baby again, spoke only gibberish and could not control his bowels and bladder. Before her husband became comatose in the veteran's hospital in Kansas, she said, "I can still tell there's a person in there. He can communicate with his eyes and gestures." During the last phase before his death, she said he was "curled up in the fetal position sucking his thumb," like the pictures we've seen of babies in their mothers' wombs.

Now, therapists and scientists at the Tavistock Institute in London, an institute that has worked with mothers and babies, *has posed the following question about people with Alzheimer's disease: "Just because they cannot communicate in a way that is comprehensible to us, can we justifiably presume that they no longer understand or have emotions?"*[1]

The Tavistock, as it is fondly called, seems to be speaking for my aunt and all the other caregivers of people with Alzheimer's. They express an emerging scientific point of view that Alzheimer's patients, like babies who cry and speak gibberish, have feelings, emotions, and a wish to communicate. Even though much of the former adult self may have disappeared because of decaying memory, those of us who have lived with and taken care of people with Alzheimer's have sensed a myriad of emotions. The irrational fears of the Alzheimer's patient who screams "get away from me" or "get out of my house" are like the fears of a child who cannot be convinced there is not a child-eating monster under his bed.

❧

B y the mid 1970s, many researchers suspected that Alzheimer's might be caused by an accumulation of aluminum in the brain. A researcher in Canada discovered aluminum in the neurofibrillary tangles that are characteristic of the disease. His published findings generated other research; some confirmed the aluminum hypothesis, but some did not.

My mother was the first one to call my attention to the aluminum connection. She told me she'd heard it on TV. "You have to stop using aluminum frying pans," she said. "And don't wrap anything in foil either. And I don't like

---

[1] Ng, Audrey V., *Making sense of dementia using infant observation techniques: a psychoanalytic perspective on a neuropathological disease.* INFANT OBSERVATION: The International Journal of Infant Observation and Its Applications, Volume 12, Number 1, April, 2009, London: The Tavistock Clinic, p. 85.

plastic. Get some of that heavy paper like the meat was wrapped in when we had our beef packaged at Denzil's."

For the next several years, friends and relatives sent me copies of newspaper and magazine articles about the possible link between aluminum and Alzheimer's. Perhaps they thought the disease had already struck and I was unable to comprehend the hubbub in the news about the possible correlation, or maybe they just wanted me to know they were thinking about me because they knew I was bumping up against the age of onset in our family. The aluminum hypothesis enjoyed incredible longevity, despite much contradictory research. By the late 1980s, one poll indicated that 33 percent of respondents believed aluminum causes Alzheimer's.

We did as Mother suggested. We stopped using aluminum pans for cooking and wrapped leftovers in paper. It would be wonderful if these simple steps kept me from getting Alzheimer's.

In the meantime, my sister was becoming more forgetful. So her husband, Scott, went a step further than giving up aluminum. He took my sister for chelation treatments. Chelation, administered intravenously, had been used successfully to treat lead poisoning and uranium exposure. In theory, the chelating agents bonded with the heavy metal ions in the blood so the harmful metals were excreted in the urine along with the water-soluble agents.

I wondered how extensive my exposure to aluminum had been. How contaminated was I? I didn't know how long we had been using aluminum cooking utensils. I remembered my sister and I used to play with pieces of used foil. Foil was interesting to crinkle and smooth out, and we used it to make miniature sculptures. Then I remembered something that sent a chill through me. The irrigation pipe on our farm had been made of aluminum. How many times had I taken a drink of water that had flowed through that aluminum pipe? Hundreds, maybe thousands.

On the farm, when we irrigated and moved the pipe to a new strip of land, the pipe left a light-color residue on my hands. Probably aluminum molecules. I often rested the pipe against my chest to make it easier to carry. Sometimes I didn't wear a shirt. Not only had I drunk water from aluminum pipe and absorbed aluminum through the skin on my hands, but through my chest.

I sat down to figure things out. We had a half mile of aluminum sprinkler pipe and a half mile of main pipe without sprinklers. Dad and I carried sixty to eighty feet of sprinkler pipe forty-five feet each carry. We moved the pipe three times a day. We did this approximately 125 days a year. I did it for eight years before I got married and left the farm. That meant I walked about 1,022 miles with my hands and sometimes my chest rubbing off aluminum particles that I might have absorbed through my skin. And this didn't count the times we loaded and unloaded the pipe on the truck to move it to a different field, or to bring it in for storage in the fall, and then to take it back to the field in the spring. If aluminum caused Alzheimer's, it was a wonder I had a brain cell left.

My sister's chelation treatments to eliminate toxic metals showed some benefit, at least initially. Immediately following the treatments, her memory and mood brightened. But by the time I decided I should be taking chelation too, the positive results proved to be temporary, and perhaps psychosomatic. My sister and her husband stopped the treatments.

In high school, my second son, Jeff, became interested in science. On the recommendation of Rita and me, he decided to attend Oberlin College in Ohio where he majored in biology. Oberlin required all students to study a topic of special interest during winter term, the month between first and second semesters. In 1980, when he was junior, he arranged to study with Leopold Liss, a neurologist at Ohio State University in Columbus who was studying Alzheimer's disease. Dr. Liss was very interested in the possible connection between Alzheimer's and aluminum in the brain.

I'd never tried to hide my concern about Alzheimer's from my children. Jeff's decision to study it during winter term was a powerful indication of his own level of concern. Jeff was engaged and was planning to get married the next summer. He was at the same stage of his life I'd been at during that summer when Artie Evans got so angry at Dad for leaving wheat stalks standing in the field.

After studying with Dr. Liss, Jeff wrote a paper and made a table of the symptoms of Alzheimer's by stages. He called the earliest stage "preclinical" and described people in this stage as "forgetful; (displaying) deviations from normal behavior patterns that have been earlier attributed to preoccupation, stress, or a temporary condition."

He sent me a copy of his paper. It arrived when I was having problems managing the Maidstone Arms. That winter—the first winter we realized we had to be open year round in order to make the inn profitable—there were thirty-one plumbing breaks in the restaurant after the first night the temperature dipped near zero. I'd tried to prevent this from happening by wrapping the pipes, but I'd failed miserably. I worried that this was comparable to the difficulty my dad experienced putting the combine together the year before I left home.

This was also the period when I took measures to help me keep track of the details of the business—notes, telephone log books, scrupulous records, you name it. Maybe Jeff had used me as the model for the first stage of Alzheimer's. I complimented my son on a great paper without mentioning I felt like its "preclinical" inspiration.

After her husband died and throughout the 1970s, Aunt Ester May expressed her faith that God had put an end to Alzheimer's in our family. "Look at the next generation," she said. "Teachers, preachers, Ph.Ds, so many of them doing such great work. God has such wonderful work for our family. I don't believe He will let this disease go on."

In the generation following Dad's, my sister was the oldest child of an affected parent. Aunt Ester May was as devastated as my mother on the day my sister started for town, as she had done an average of twice a week for forty years, arrived at U.S. Highway 270, three-quarters of a mile from the house, and couldn't remember whether to turn right or left. No matter how she approached the question, she couldn't decide, so she turned around and went home. She never drove again. My sister had been afraid for a long time she was getting Alzheimer's, but that was the day she knew for sure.

Ester May immediately admitted she had been wrong; no one, she said, can read the mind of God. God didn't intend to stop the disease with Uncle George and my father's generation. If one person, my sister, could get it, any of us could get it, including her own children. Ester May revised her faith. "God expects us, yes us, to do something about it," she said, "and we had better get busy."

Since the early 1970s, Ester May had been speaking to a young Christian research scientist named Gary Miner. Gary and his wife, Linda, were Nazarenes, a group formed from the holiness tradition with which Ester May's father, a farmer and preacher, had been affiliated. Their common faith was important to Aunt Ester May. She still believed that faith in God was the only hope for finding a cure for our family's problem.

Ester May tracked down and teamed up with two other people whose families had Familial Early Onset Alzheimer's Disease, and the three contacted everyone they could find with an interest in the familial form of Alzheimer's.

Ester May persuaded Robert Cook, a doctor at the University of Colorado, to study our family. After she organized educational meetings for the family, researchers began collecting blood and skin samples from those of us who were willing to give them.

Dr. Cook tried to get funding for the research but was unsuccessful. Exhausted by the effort he'd expended to study Alzheimer's disease, he left the university for a position in Washington. The research program at Colorado limped forward one more year, but with no ongoing funds, it eventually fizzled out. The family became a research orphan.

Ester May, however, was never idle. She continued her relationship with Gary and Linda Miner. She called them regularly, asking, "Can you help us?" Through the urgings of Ester May and the other two advocates who were trying to get help for Alzheimer's families, the Miners, using their own money and a few small grants, started the Familial Alzheimer's Disease Research Foundation. They recruited a number of well-known public figures and respected academics, and researchers to serve on the board. They cashed in their retirement funds and traveled around the country in a camper, collecting DNA samples from members of the three families, including ours. They got blood from my cousin in Ohio and my brother in Missouri, and they made several trips to visit my sister and brother-in-law on their farm in Oklahoma. The Miners set up their camper at our farm and asked family members to come have blood drawn.

The Miners designed a sophisticated "neuropsychological risk facture study,"[2] a test to predict which family members would develop Alzheimer's. They administered the test to anyone in line for the gene who wanted to participate. They emphasized that the test was for research purposes only, and they had no plans to share their predictions. That was fine with my family; no one wanted to know if they were going to get the disease.

Meanwhile, Ester May had been in touch with the U.S. Senators and Representatives from Oklahoma and had talked to them about our family problem. Congress had become interested in Alzheimer's disease, both the rare early onset Alzheimer's, which afflicted our family, and the more common later onset Alzheimer's called sporadic Alzheimer's. Ester May was invited to testify at congressional hearings. She told the assembled politicians how Alzheimer's had disrupted our lives and brought some family members to the brink of bankruptcy.

As a result of the hearings, Congress became convinced that Alzheimer's disease, considered a rare affliction when it was diagnosed in Uncle George and my father, was, in fact, a major health problem with devastating effects on the lives of many Americans. Legislators began working to establish Alzheimer's Disease Research Centers throughout the country to address what would soon become an epidemic when the postwar baby boomers reached retirement and the average age of death continued to rise.

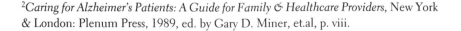

---

[2] *Caring for Alzheimer's Patients: A Guide for Family & Healthcare Providers*, New York & London: Plenum Press, 1989, ed. by Gary D. Miner, et.al, p. viii.

Even after Dr. Cook and his fellow University of Colorado researchers took blood samples from some members of our family, many of my relatives continued to find the thought of blood research unnerving, nearly unthinkable.

So when Gary Miner and Dr. Thomas Bird, a neurologist from Seattle with a sub-specialty in genetic diseases, set out from Tulsa to gather samples from our family, they had their work cut out for them.

Dr. Bird was part of the University of Washington's Alzheimer's Disease Research Center, along with Dr. George Martin, who studied aging and diseases of aging. Alzheimer's disease is a disease of aging because it appears more frequently as the average age of the population increases.

Dr. Bird had been studying hereditary neuropathy, a disease that causes weakness of the hands and feet. He analyzed the DNA of people with the disease to identify the chromosome containing the disease-causing gene, hoping someday to isolate the gene itself. Martin and Bird combined their interests and experiences and designed a research project to study the genetics of familial early onset Alzheimer's disease. Since the plaques and tangles found in the brains of people with Alzheimer's occurred whether people died with the disease in their fortiess or their eighties, they theorized that the early onset Alzheimer's, although rarer than sporadic Alzheimer's, might hold the key to finding treatments for both types. The search was to be conducted by Gerard Schellenberg, Ph.D., a Neurogeneticist.

After their application was funded, the Seattle ADRC began looking for families with early onset Alzheimer's. Dr. Bird in Seattle contacted Dr. Miner in Tulsa who told him about Ester May and our family. The car trip that began in Tulsa resulted from that contact.

Dr. Miner had anticipated that funding for the national Alzheimer's Disease Research Centers might trigger a demand for DNA from our family. Now that awareness and concern about Alzheimer's had exploded into the public consciousness, it was likely that those who unlocked the key to prevention and treatment would, someday, win the Nobel Prize. Understanding the competitive nature of researchers, Dr. Miner encouraged our family to require all blood seekers to sign an agreement promising to share their research material and progress with one other. It was a fortuitous move given how competitive the search for genes would become within the scientific community.

Dr. Bird and Dr. Miner first stopped in Clinton, located west of Oklahoma City on Route 66. Uncle Otto lay in the veterans' hospital in Clinton, curled in a fetal position, just like Frau Auguste D, Dr. Alzheimer's patient, had been described when she lay in her bed in Frankfurt, Germany, eighty years earlier. Aunt Marie had given permission for the doctors to draw my uncle's blood. Since my uncle was comatose, there would be no resistance at this stop.

The doctors then made another stop in Clinton, at the home of my father's youngest brother, Delmer, now in his mid-fifties and in the throes of Alzheimer's. Soft-spoken Aunt Marie had promised strident Aunt Ester May that she'd ask Delmer and his wife to cooperate, talk to the doctors, and give blood, if only for the sake of Marie and Otto's children, who were like younger siblings to their Uncle Delmer because he had stayed with the family when he went to college.

The doctors' third call that day was in Lawton, sixty miles south, where my cousin Darold was a physician. There should be no problem getting blood from him. He knew the importance of research. He knew how his mother had suffered.

However, Darold had children of his own. He worried that by becoming a research subject he might magnify his children's fear of Alzheimer's. He didn't want to create a storm cloud over their future before anything could be done about the problem. But in the end, he gave his consent and gave his blood.

One year later, Dr. Miner and Aunt Ester May held a meeting in the First Christian Church in my hometown. Through the resources of the foundation he and his wife, Linda, had started, Dr. Miner persuaded some of the best researchers in the world to journey to this remote Oklahoma panhandle town to share the research they were doing with each other and with our family.

Dr. Bird flew in from Seattle. Although he was surprised and pleased that so many well-known scientists were gathering in such a remote locale to share their results, Dr. Bird was disappointed that there were no people at the meeting with symptoms of the disease. He still had only the two samples gathered the year before from my uncles Otto and Delmer. The number of samples from affected people was inadequate for serious research. Dr. Bird didn't know he was about to stumble on the mother lode.

After the meeting, he visited Aunt Ester May, hoping to obtain some background information about our family, which he'd add to the information he already had about other families involved in the research at the fledgling Alzheimer's Disease Research Center in Seattle. He asked Ester May about our family's ethnic background. She hesitated. She knew the family had made great efforts since the outbreak of World War I to avoid the prejudices of rural independent western America toward both Germans and Russians. We had said we were Dutch so often we almost believed it.

But this time, Ester told the truth, based on the information she'd collected while tracing the family tree to find out who had Alzheimer's. The Reiswigs are Volga Germans, she told Dr. Bird. Our family left Germany a long time ago and spent more than a hundred years living along the Volga River in Russia.

When my aunt said, "Volga Germans," a lightbulb went on in Dr. Bird's head. He asked her to repeat what she had just said. Then he said the members of another family he'd enlisted in his research, a family from the west coast and Alaska, had described themselves as Volga Germans. In fact, he said, a family member had written a book called *The Volga Pilgrims*.

Ester May told Dr. Bird she knew of two other families with early onset Alzheimer's who came to North America from the same area in Russia, west of the Volga River.

Dr. Bird returned to Seattle certain he had stumbled on some important information. He and the other researchers doubled back and re-interviewed all the families they had identified with familial early onset Alzheimer's. They determined that about half of the families were Volga Germans. Eventually, they found eleven Volga German families with familial early onset Alzheimer's disease. Ten of the families were from two villages west of the Volga, Walter and Frank, only seven miles apart, and the eleventh was from Norka, a village ten miles from Walter.

Dr. Bird was confident he had discovered a unique set of research subjects with a common ancestor, a founder. He believed one ancestor of all these families had left Germany with the group who departed from Hesse near Frankfurt and arrived at the Volga in 1766.

Furthermore, he theorized, it was highly possible that Frau Auguste D, the patient Dr. Alzhiemer began treating in 1901, was a distant relative of these Volga Germans, because she lived in Frankfurt, their homeland, and her symptoms and age of onset were so similar to what he was now finding in the Volga German families in North America.

$$\textit{\textbf{\aa}}$$

The theory that aluminum caused Alzheimer's persisted into the early 1990s. But doubts grew. In 1995, Duke University conducted a study of Alzheimer's patients that concluded there was "no consistent relationship between aluminum in the body and Alzheimer's disease."[3] Rita and I began using aluminum foil to wrap food once again.

Meanwhile, researchers had made no progress in their search for a gene that caused Alzheimer's. Then, in 1991, *The New York Times* ran the headline: GENE MUTATION THAT CAUSES ALZHEIMER'S IS FOUND. Researchers in England and the United States had found a gene on Chromosome 21, which they called APP, short for amyloid precursor

---

[3]Pierce, Charles P., *Hard to Forget*, New York: Random House, 2000, p. 48.

protein. These researchers had been looking for an Alzheimer's gene on chromosome 21 because the Down syndrome gene was located there. Both people with Down syndrome and people with Alzheimer's have excess amyloid protein in their bodies; researchers weren't sure if this was a cause or result of the disease.

When I saw the article, my heart beat faster. There seemed to be wide agreement that this was the Alzheimer's gene for the early onset type of the disease. Now the effort to find treatments could begin.

However, within a few days, I received disappointing news from Seattle: this mutation wasn't present in the Volga Germans' DNA. Our disease had another cause. There had to be another gene. Soon other researchers weighed in. Not only did the mutation on chromosome 21 not account for the Washington research subjects, it did not apply to many other early onset cases. Eventually researchers would learn that the mutation on chromosome 21 accounted for only two percent of early onset Alzheimer's.

The search for another location was on even before the discovery of the gene on chromosome 21 was announced. The University of Washington team began sifting through chromosome 14, and in June 1992 they detected a flaw, although they didn't pinpoint its precise location. Three years later, Rudolph Tanzi, a professor of neurology in Boston, and his team of researchers pinpointed the defective gene on chromosome 14. This gene, called Presenilin 1, affected more people than APP; it accounted for nearly thirty percent of all early onset Alzheimer's cases. But the Volga German families in the University of Washington study were not among them.

About two weeks after the official announcement of Presenilin 1's precise location on chromosome 14, Rudolph Tanzi talked to Dr. Schellenberg, who was part of the University of Washington scientific team. The two were colleagues, as close to being friends as rivals can be. Schellenberg was discouraged. His team seemed to be on the wrong track in their search for the Volga German gene. Although Tanzi had access to a frozen Volga German brain in the freezer at Massachusetts General Hospital and could have searched for the gene himself, Tanzi told Schellenberg his lab had noted a homolog (a similar gene) of the mutated gene on chromosome 14, somewhere on the long arm of chromosome 1 "Maybe that's your Volga German gene," he suggested. Chromosome 1 is the longest of all the chromosomes, making it the most difficult to search. Schellenberg was skeptical about Tanzi's suggestion. Nevertheless, he began the search.

Chapter Eleven

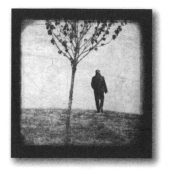

THE MIRACLE

*A*fter the mutation on the gene *called APP was identified and located on chromosome 21, and it was determined the gene was not the problem that affected our family—that it, in fact, only affected about two percent of early onset cases—it was four long years before more news about early onset genes surfaced. Those were years my wife and I stood on high alert, watching for symptoms of Alzheimer's to occur in me. Every small incident of forgetfulness or poor judgment might be a sign. Then the news hit. A new mutation causing early onset Alzheimer's had been traced to chromosome 14. Scientists named it Presenilin 1. There were, in fact, more than forty different mutations in the Presenilin 1 gene causing Alzheimer's to strike as early as age twenty-eight and as late as sixty-two, with an average age of onset in the mid-forties. Like APP, Presenilin 1 is involved in protein production. The mutations elevate levels of beta amyloid in the blood and brains of people who carry the defective gene. This gene*

affects many more people than APP, more than thirty percent of
early onset cases according to most estimates.

The research team at the ADRC in Seattle working with our
DNA, and the DNA of other Volga German families, had helped
in the process of locating the area on chromosome 14 where the
mutations occurred, but Doctors Bird and Schellenberg knew these
anomalies were not present in our DNA. Presenilin 1 was not our
defective gene.

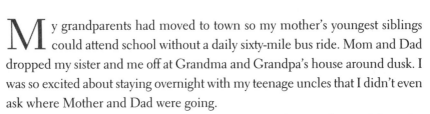

My grandparents had moved to town so my mother's youngest siblings could attend school without a daily sixty-mile bus ride. Mom and Dad dropped my sister and me off at Grandma and Grandpa's house around dusk. I was so excited about staying overnight with my teenage uncles that I didn't even ask where Mother and Dad were going.

We were having breakfast the next morning when Dad arrived from the hospital with the news that our mother had given birth to a baby boy. He grew tall, was blond, quiet, athletic. My mother adored him.

My sister was popular in high school. She was the football queen in her freshman year. She dated the star linebacker. The summer after her graduation, she married a young man in our church, a farmer's son. After their wedding, they lived in town and started their family, which would grow to include three boys and a girl. When Mother knew it was time to turn over the farm, my sister and her husband were ready to take charge. Her family was my mother's anchor.

My sister stopped driving about fifteen years after Dad died. Mother watched in horror as her daughter's health declined. My sister's eyes sunk back behind her brows and became black opaque pools. Her spark—the spark that got her crowned football queen and kept her just as popular as an adult— slowly dimmed. When visitors came, she sat in a recliner with her feet off the floor, staring straight ahead, sometimes rocking back and forth.

One night she woke up and began screaming at her husband to get away from her. If he didn't get out of the room, she warned, she'd kill him. She thought he was a stranger who had crept into bed with her.

My sister was a gentle person by nature; the kitchen knife was the only thing she'd used to kill anything. As Mother had taught us, she strung chickens from the clothesline by their feet with a piece of binder twine, grabbed them by the neck, cut off their heads, and left the flapping birds to turn pink with their own blood. Her husband knew she couldn't string him up from the clothes-line, but he was afraid she might, in a fit of panic and rage, try to cut off his head. After that night, he hid the kitchen knives.

Soon, even with help from Mother and others, my brother-in-law could no longer care for my sister, and he put her in the local nursing home.

When he grew up, my brother became the tallest member of our family. He was also the smartest. He graduated high school first in his class.

In college, he majored in music. He then joined the Navy band as a French horn player. He later played for the Kansas City and St. Louis symphonies.

When the St. Louis symphony played a concert at Carnegie Hall, Mother came to New York and we both attended. During a break between pieces, she turned to me and said, "Our boy is so handsome, isn't he?" She always called him "our boy."

When he was about forty, my brother forgot to pay the household bills. He made excuses to his wife, claiming he just hadn't have time to get to them, but she immediately began to worry. She knew about the Alzheimer's gene. She took over the family finances.

One day a few years later, my brother dropped his wife at the grocery store and then took their daughter to her ballet lesson nearby. Then he somehow wound up on the interstate highway. He was gone nearly two hours before he found his way back to the grocery store, where his wife was waiting, panicked.

He continued driving for some time after this episode, often making his passengers uneasy by improvising his own road rules, such as making left turns from the right lane.

Then one day, his wife told him his driving had gotten too dangerous; he had to stop. My brother left the house in a rage. When he returned, hours later, he handed her his keys and told her he knew she was right. He never drove again.

My brother had been playing the horn since he was in the ninth grade, and for all of his professional life. Even after he began to decline, he still could play, as long he was familiar with the music. But when he had to read music and follow cues, he got lost.

His last job was with a small symphony in Kentucky. When the director asked him to resign, my brother asked, "What am I going to do with myself?"

He took a job as the custodian at his family's church. When he could no longer track what needed to be done, the church made him assistant custodian so someone else could remind him of what he forgot.

When my brother could no longer play music but could still carry on a conversation, he, his wife, and their two daughters came to visit us in East

Hampton He and I went for a walk through the village, playing a game we'd played as kids when Dad drove us to church each Sunday: identifying the make and model of the cars we passed.

Although he'd been officially diagnosed with early stage Alzheimer's disease, my brother was still very good at this game. Better at it than I was.

By now, at age fifty-five, I'd started thinking that, perhaps, the Alzheimer's gene had skipped me. But it was by no means a sure thing. The age of onset varied widely, as illustrated by Uncle Otto, whose symptoms began in his early fifties, and my Uncle George whose symptoms began in his late thirties. I still worried whenever I went to the basement and forgot why, or when I misplaced my keys, or when I couldn't remember an acquaintance's name.

During our walk, my brother identified a Ferrari and an Aston Martin and could tell the difference between a Bentley and a Rolls Royce. I only knew General Motors, Chrysler, and Ford, and I even confused those a few times. I thought, "If my brother has Alzheimer's, I've got it, too. I'm obviously more advanced than he is, but I don't even know it. Not knowing must be a symptom of the disease."

Later that afternoon, while we were sitting in the kitchen, my brother told me he wanted to go to his room and lie down. I said okay. He paused and then said, "I don't know where the room is."

My brother and his wife were staying in an apartment above our garage, just a few feet from the kitchen door. I pointed and said, "Go out the door and then into the next door. Turn left up the steps, and you're there."

He walked to the screen door and pushed, but it didn't open. He didn't notice the door latch. He hesitated, confused. I just sat and watched; I was afraid to intrude, but I was also curious to see what he'd do.

What he did was inexplicable. He tried to climb out the window but his shoulders were too broad to fit through. As I watched him, I felt dizzy. What had I been thinking, worrying about myself when my younger brother—"our boy"—was unable to find his way out the door.

I got out of my seat, opened the door, and led him by the hand, as I had led my father and grandfather.

◢

On Friday, after my brother and his family headed home to the Midwest, I settled down to read the newspaper. On an inside page, a headline caught my eye: THIRD GENE TIED TO EARLY ONSET ALZHEIMER'S. The article began: "A gene mutation found among a small group with German-Russian ancestry has been identified as the third to cause early onset Alzheimer's disease. Scientists say the discovery may speed the development of drugs to combat the disorder." [1]

I knew the article was about us.

The story referred to a longer article scheduled to appear that day in *Science* magazine. I found a copy of *Science* so I could read it. When I opened the magazine, there was our family tree, going all the way back to my great-great grandfather, who came to the United States from Russia. Dad and nine of his siblings were represented with black circles and squares, signifying that they had the gene. In my generation, my white square stood between the black circle of my sister and the black square of my brother.

The article confirmed what I had always hoped: I didn't have the gene. I wouldn't get early onset Alzheimer's.

At first, I was overwhelmed with relief and elation. I wanted to sing. But those feelings of intense happiness were soon mitigated by guilt and grief. Why had I escaped when both my sister and brother had not?

◢

Now that researchers had located the gene, they could begin the difficult process of finding potential treatments and cures. It was too late for our generation; the discovery couldn't reverse my siblings' fate. But maybe it wasn't too late for our children.

---

[1] *The New York Times*, Friday, August 18, 1995.

No, not "our children." My children no longer would be haunted by this danger. I meant "their children," my brother's and sister's kids, and the children of my cousins who have a parent affected by the disease.

For me, and for my children, the nightmare was over. I merely had to live with my legacy of guilt and grief.

Chapter Twelve

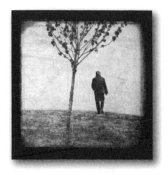

THE UNLUCKY BEAUTY

Late onset Alzheimer's, arbitrarily denoted as onset after age sixty-five, has no obvious inheritance pattern that has been found. Except one gene has been found that has been termed the "susceptibility" gene: ApoE on chromosome 19. The ApoE gene comes in several different forms, or alleles, but three occur most frequently: E2, E3, and E4. We all inherit one allele from each parent. E2 alleles appear to lower the risk for getting Alzheimer's, E3s appear to be neutral, and one E4 allele doubles the risk while two E4s increases the risk by about eight to ten times.

In my family, E4s are common. My dad's oldest brother who did not have Presenilin 2, the gene in our family that causes early onset, had obvious symptoms of Alzheimer's by age sixty-eight and died totally senile at seventy-eight. He had two copies of E4. Every family member whose blood was tested as part of the Seattle study published in 1995 has at least one copy of E4, including myself.

My family has a genetic risk for not only early onset Alzheimer's disease from Presenilin 1 with its dominant fifty-fifty risk, but has a gene increasing the likelihood of having the late onset form of the disease.

Fortunately, it is starting to appear that late onset Alzheimer's, and the specific age it strikes people, is much more affected by environmental factors than the early onset type. Those of us with one or two ApoE4s do not have to be passive victims. More and more proof is coming in. We have it within our own power to modify, to one degree or another, our futures. Science tells us: what's good for the heart is good for the brain.

***

"Don't think this will be pretty," my Aunt Marie said, as we drove across town toward the nursing home.

I hadn't seen my cousin Anne for a few years. She had been in her forties then, and working at a convenience store, clerking and making simple sandwiches from behind a counter. At the time, Uncle Otto was still alive and lay curled up in the Veteran's Hospital in Clinton. One day Aunt Marie had asked me to drive Anne into the rough rangeland north of the river where Anne's husband, a carpenter, was working on a ranch house. He'd called Anne and asked her to bring him some supplies.

I was suspicious when my aunt asked for my help; she rarely asked anyone to do anything for her. After we returned to Marie's house, and my cousin Anne went home, Marie cornered me and asked if I thought her daughter was getting Alzheimer's. I had noticed some unusual hesitancy and moments of confusion. I tried to both tell her what I saw and reassure her, but she could not hold back her tears.

When we entered Anne's room in the nursing home, she was out of bed and sitting up in a large chair. A nurse had combed her hair, but it was flattened on one side and looked unwashed. Anne's head was tilted. Aunt Marie bent over her and spoke in that voice people use to speak to foreigners—loud and slow. "Anne, your cousin Gary is here to see you. You know Gary. You remember Gary." There was no life in her eyes, just a continuous "thousand mile stare."

Anne slid sideways in her chair. "I don't know why she's so bent over this way," Aunt Marie said. I remembered that my sister's spine bent in the same direction. I stepped behind my cousin's chair to help. Her neck, her whole spinal column was rigid. We couldn't straighten her, so we propped her up with pillows.

"Every day I think 'I can't do this anymore,'" Marie said quietly. "But then at 4:30 I come over." As she spoke, an aide brought Anne's dinner. It consisted of one course: a white, creamlike substance. The aide put a towel around my cousin's neck. Aunt Marie picked up the spoon.

"Here's your dinner, darling," she said, and touched the spoon to my cousin's lips. Anne opened her mouth just enough so my aunt could pour in half a spoonful of the white stuff. The rest ran down her chin. Marie wiped it off with the towel.

"When the staff feeds her, they use a turkey baster and squirt the food," Aunt Marie told me. "I hate that. Sometimes she chokes." Marie added, "She's living on hardly anything, but look how large she is."

It was true. Anne was tall, like my Uncle Otto, and she'd always been more solid than skinny. But now she was heavier. Otto had shrunk to seventy-one pounds on a feeding tube, but a few milligrams of white superfood kept his daughter physically robust despite her bent spine and blank demeanor.

The feeding took twenty minutes. Then an aide came to take away the tray. I watched my aunt for cues. She was ready to go. We said good-bye to Anne, and Anne said nothing in response.

As we walked down the hall, the smells of disinfectant and the sounds of patients were all too familiar to me. Around the corner from my cousin's room was the room where my sister had lived in an Alzheimer's stupor for six years. My mother's room was on this same hall.

Following her first stroke, Mother had a series of smaller stokes. She couldn't speak. One day when I was reading to her at the nursing home, Aunt Ester May came into the room. I stood up to accept Ester May's bone-crushing hug and chatted with her for a moment. Then I turned to see my mother's eyes flash, her face grimace, and her lips purse as she squeezed out two perfectly pronounced words, clearly aimed in Ester May's direction: "Go home!"

Mother uttered only one other word during her months in the nursing home. As I was pushing her in her wheelchair down the hall one afternoon, she suddenly said, "Barn." Or that's what it sounded like.

I stopped walking and knelt down in front of her thin, bent figure. "Did you say 'barn'?" I asked. Mother nodded.

I leaned back against the wall and laughed. Mother started laughing, too. I don't know how long it had been since we'd laughed together—how long since there'd been anything to laugh about. But once we started, we couldn't stop. And it was contagious. Two nurses stopped beside us and began to laugh too. Then some visitors started in. I couldn't tell anyone what was so funny. In truth, we were laughing—so hard that tears ran down our cheeks—because things were so sad.

The nursing home, with its odors of adult diapers and soiled linens and disinfectant, smelled like the barn after we washed the cows' udders with disinfectant and attached the milking machines to their teats. In her view, Mother was living in, and would die in, the barn.

As Aunt Marie and I walked down that same hall after visiting Anne, she said, "I can't stand to see my child this way. I'll miss her so much when she's gone. But this is too much—too long. I wish the Lord would take her. And now there's. . . ."

She stopped before saying her son's name. I knew she would cry if she said it.

Karl was once a skilled carpenter and cabinetmaker like Uncle Otto. But he'd just lost his last job, as a custodian at a hobby shop. Within a year, he'd be in a nursing home like this one.

My aunt and I sat at a table at the Cactus Grill. We'd both filled our plates at the all-you-can-eat salad bar. I splurged on chicken-fried steak.

After we left the nursing home, our mood lightened. We were almost jovial. We kept our conversation in the present tense, talking about the food and the people who stopped by our table to say hello. I watched Aunt Marie as she ate. She was impeccably dressed, and her black hair, now mostly gray, was carefully styled. She was still a beautiful woman.

The tough, gristly texture of my chicken-fried steak was so familiar; it was the same meal I'd had on Friday nights in high school, after football games. If Rita were here, she'd chide me about my unhealthy eating habits. But I felt as if I were living on bonus time. And what's bonus time worth if you don't enjoy it?

As I ate, I reflected on my aunt's life, a Grimm's fairy tale in two parts. In the first part, she married a tall, handsome man, bore two beautiful children, and lived in a comfortable home her husband had built with his own hands, furnished with antiques she'd refinished herself. She had many close, loving relatives and dear friends.

Then came the second part of the tale, the plot of which was determined by a series of genetic coin tosses. First, her husband, then her daughter, and then her son fell victim to Alzheimer's. Aunt Marie and her family lost the coin toss three times out of three.

Marie now had four grandsons and a growing brood of great grandchildren. "I wish they'd stop having children," she said to me one day. She didn't have to explain what she meant.

Maybe the law of averages would catch up, and her grandsons would be spared the family disease. But a coin toss is arbitrary. No matter how many times the coin comes up tails, there's a fifty-fifty chance it will be tails again next time.

Chapter Thirteen

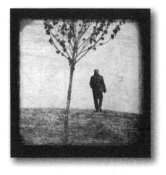

THE MAN WHO
WANTED TO KNOW

I *contacted all my relatives I could*
track down to tell them I was writing a book about our family. I
invited them to talk about their experiences dealing with our fam-
ily's inherited Alzheimer's disease. One of my cousins whom I have
never met replied and asked if I knew of any research she could be
part of that might help science come up with treatments and a cure
for the disease. She is in her mid-forties, a daughter of my dad's
younger sister, Ruby, who died in her fifties with Alzheimer's. With
my family's average age of onset bearing down on her, my cousin
admitted she is afraid as she faces the genetic coin flip. Another
cousin, Chuck, had signed up to participate in a study called DIAN
(Dominantly Inherited Alzheimer's Network), so I told her about it.

DIAN will study 300 volunteers whose parents have (or had,
if dead) one of the three identified familial early onset Alzheimer's

genes, APP, PS1, or PS2. The National Institute on Aging has provided funding for the sixteen million dollar study that unites ten separate research agencies in the U.S., the UK, and Australia. One initial goal is to establish a patient registry for those children of affected parents, children who now face a fifty-percent risk of having early onset Alzheimer's.

Participants are asked to undergo several rigorous procedures, including brain scans (PIB-PET amyloid imaging), blood analysis, and a spinal fluid sample that requires a lumbar puncture. These procedures will help achieve DIAN's main goal: to understand how Alzheimer's develops in the decade before symptoms are noticed, so that, eventually, treatment can begin even before symptoms appear.

Most scientists believe that the process of developing Alzheimer's is the same for both early and late onset. The DIAN study has as its eventual goal the development of therapies for both types beginning before the emergence of symptoms.

O n the day after Christmas, 2007, *The New York Times* published the sixth of a series of front-page articles called "Six Killers." The first five articles covered heart disease, cancer, stroke, chronic obstructive pulmonary disease, and diabetes. The sixth article was entitled "Finding Alzheimer's Before a Mind Fails."

The article included a link to a website that contained video reports about Alzheimer's. I went to the site and clicked on a picture of two clasped hands. A title appeared: "The Rarest Gene." This startled me.

Of the Alzheimer's genes that have been found so far, the one that afflicts my family is the rarest, afflicting only about 200 known people. The video had to be about our Volga German gene.

A man's voice came over the opening credits: "I'm not afraid of dying. At the most, I'm afraid of living too long, where I can't decide for myself what I want to do about things." His voice was like that of a Baptist preacher, rich and resonant. But he hesitated before every second or third word, struggling to find a way to express what he wanted to say. It was a speech pattern familiar to me from my dad, my uncles and aunts, and my sister and brother.

Then the speaker's face appeared on my computer screen. I recognized my cousin Chuck, the youngest son of Dad's sister, Reba. I hadn't seen him since his mother's funeral in 1973, but I recognized him immediately.

Before I could recover from my shock at seeing my cousin, Chuck did the unthinkable. He held up a portrait of the fourteen brothers and sisters in our parents' generation. I was at the photography studio with Dad when the picture was taken, back in the late 1950s, in Perryton, Texas. It was the last time all fourteen siblings got together.

While Chuck spoke, the camera zoomed in on the old photo. He pointed and said, "This one had Alzheimer's . . . this one had Alzheimer's . . . and this one." I held my breath as I watched. I both did and didn't want him to point to Dad.

The camera zoomed even closer and focused on Chuck's mother. "My mother . . . she had Alzheimer's." Now his voice quavered and labored with sorrow.

Although the photograph was in black and white, I could see Chuck's mother in the vivid Kelly greens and purples she often wore to complement her deep red hair.

As I watched Chuck talk about our family, my first thought was this: He's outed us. He's outed the family. Boy, will everyone be mad. But that thought faded fast.

Now I know—and my family knows—that Chuck's revelation came not a moment too soon. Our family had spoken barely a word about the disease since my Aunt Ester May testified before Congress more than twenty years ago. It was time to talk, and the more people who talked, the better.

I settled my mind enough to listen to the rest of the video. Dr. Thomas Bird began speaking about how the Volga German connection was unearthed and how some of its mysteries were solved.

Then Chuck reappeared and told a story about his mother. One summer day, nearly forty years ago, Chuck was plowing a field on their farm. When he took a break for a drink of water, he noticed his mother wasn't in the house. Chuck went outside to look for her. It hadn't rained for a few weeks; he found footprints in the dust and followed them down the road. The prints led to a small, dry creek that ran under the road, through a steel culvert, a few hundred feet from the house. At the entrance of the culvert, Chuck found his mother's clothes.

He was a young teenager. He didn't know what to do. His shoulders barely fit in the culvert's opening—there was just enough room for him to worm himself in. He finally reached his mother in the middle of the culvert, six feet under the road. When he asked her what she was doing there, she begged him to leave her alone and let her die.

Chuck edged himself out of the culvert and ran back to the house to grab a blanket. He crawled back into the culvert and, and inch by inch pulled her out, wrapped her in the blanket, and brought her back to the house.

But she still wanted to die, and she asked Chuck to help her. He told her he couldn't. At that point, however, he stopped praying for her recovery and started praying for her death. In the video, he said, "There's a lot of guilt . . . that at some point you'd prefer someone to die rather than continue to go through that kind of anguish and pain."

Then Chuck spoke about getting tested for the early onset Alzheimer's gene and finding out he had it. He'd been the only member of our family to take the test.

Finally, Chuck explained why he participated in the video. "We're not going quietly to our grave with this disease. We're going to talk about it. And that's hopefully going to bring action. If not for me, at least for my daughter and the other children who are following parents with early onset."

🍃

A couple of months after I saw the video, my wife, my sons Jesse and Jeff, and Jeff's wife, Julie, made a trip to Portland, Oregon, to visit my grandson, Jaymz, and his fiancé, Amy. I also planned to see my cousin Chuck, who lived in Albany, Oregon, about fifty miles southwest of Portland.

When I pulled up at Chuck's house, I saw a beat-up pickup truck parked in front and thought, "The boy may be out of the panhandle, but the panhandle is still in the boy."

And when Chuck opened the door, I saw the face of a boy, although in fact he was fifty-three. Despite his sadness, a twinkle played in his eyes. As we shook hands and hugged, I couldn't help staring, trying both to know him and to gauge the progress of the disease. At the end of *The New York Times* video, the narrator had said, "As for Chuck, his condition has worsened. He now has trouble speaking and controlling his movements." Within thirty seconds of seeing Chuck, I knew those words were too pessimistic. The filmmakers probably wanted to give their video a satisfying narrative arc and emphasize the gravity of the disease.

As if to answer the questions he knew I had, Chuck handed me a business card that said "Ask Me About Alzheimer's Disease—Let's Talk" and identified Chuck as a "Speaker on Early Stage Issues."

We settled into a conversation in his living room. He reminded me he had an afternoon meeting at a nearby senior citizen's center; he was leading a group that gathered monthly to talk about early stage Alzheimer's. I asked if I could go with him, and he agreed.

"How's your brother?" I asked. Chuck knew which brother I was talking about. His oldest brother, Hank, was alive and well, a professor of Agronomy in Montana. Another brother, Darold, who was two years older than Chuck, had died seven years ago. When he started having trouble with his memory, he went to the Mayo Clinic and learned that he had a brain tumor. Darold was paralyzed when a doctor inserted a needle into his brain for a biopsy. He died a year later.

The brother I was asking about, Darin, was the second oldest, and was in an assisted living facility in Texas. Doctors diagnosed his Alzheimer's a few years before Chuck's. "He's at the point where he can still recognize people, and he understands words, but he can't speak," Chuck said.

I told him a little about what had happened in my family, with my dad, my sister, and my brother. We discussed early symptoms, the "early stage issues" as he phrased it on his card, when the ability to make reasonably good judgments begins to fade into questionable, then hopelessly poor, judgments. I told him about my dad dehorning our herd of registered cattle.

"Did any of your family ever run over snakes?" Chuck asked.

In the panhandle, rattlesnakes were viewed as dangerous to humans but even more dangerous to cattle, especially to young calves. Chuck told me his mother "made it her personal mission to run over every rattlesnake she saw." He said, "She chased one into the bar ditch and tore up the underneath of a nearly new car. My dad was really mad and had a talk with her. He explained she couldn't do that. One snake doesn't make that much difference. She said she understood, but the next time she saw a snake, she did it again and tore up another car. We didn't know she was getting sick. We didn't know why she couldn't use better judgment."

"When did you know about the Alzheimer's?" I asked.

"I was thirteen or fourteen," Chuck said. "After the snakes, mom started letting herself go. It really upset my dad. We knew people were talking." He continued, "And the other thing she did was just sit and stare. We called it the thousand mile stare. She forgot to do important things. If my brother and I had after-school activities and didn't come home from school to help her, she'd forget to prepare supper for my dad.

"Finally my dad called a meeting of us boys and said we had to pray. He was thinking of divorcing our mother because she had gotten so stubborn and lazy. When we talked to my mother, she told me and my brother we should go talk to Aunt Ester May. She could tell us what was wrong. Then she said, 'Just don't tell your dad.'

"As you know, Ester May had a reputation in the family, and my dad was one of them that didn't like her. Anyhow, that's when I learned about Alzheimer's."

We headed out the door to lunch. I told Chuck I'd drive my rental car so he wouldn't have to burn his gas. There was an uneasy moment when I thought he'd insist on driving his truck. "My driving's fine," he told me. I thought, "Yep, so was Granddad's, up to the moment he drove his truck onto the Huntoon crossing." Chuck relented and allowed me to drive. He'd navigate, he said. He guided me to a shopping center where there was a sandwich shop. We slid into a booth.

After we ordered, he said, "It depresses me to talk about Mom. I can't remember where I was."

"You told your Dad what Ester May said. Was he then more understanding?"

"Even after Dad seemed to accept that my mother had a disease and that's what was causing her to act the way she was, he'd go back to thinking what he thought before, that she was just stubborn, being a disobedient wife.

"When I graduated high school, I got the hell out of there. It was just too much responsibility for a young kid to take care of her. To deal with it, and to see her go down hill like she did. I hate to admit it, but I ran. Dad had to put her in the nursing home."

"We all ran," I said.

As I talked to Chuck, I felt increasingly close to him, and I realized I wanted another chance at having a younger brother, or, more specifically, at being a better older brother. I had kept myself at a distance from my brother because it was so painful to watch him go through his illness. I wanted to do things over—to stay and face it.

Later that afternoon, I started hearing the hesitation in Chuck's voice as he groped for words, as he had in the video. "He's getting tired," I thought. I remembered how that happened to my dad and my sister. They were good in the morning, and not so good later in the afternoon and evening.

Chuck told me about his first Alzheimer's symptoms, which occurred while he was working for a railroad union in Oregon.

"I went to work one morning with a black shoe on and a brown one," he said. "This was after I got tested for the gene. But I didn't think anything was wrong. I thought I was fine. No one had given me any bad reports."

"Well, it's the kind of thing that can happen," I said. "We've all done it, at least with socks."

"My boss called me in," Chuck continued. "'People are laughing at you,' she said. 'You can't maintain respect with this kind of thing. Go home and change your shoes.' So I did."

The slight hesitation in his speech now became more pronounced. I felt him drifting away. There was a little catch in his breath. "So did you go back to your office?" I asked.

He turned and looked at me. He seemed to think he'd already explained. Maybe he had, but I didn't understand.

"Yes, I went back," he said. "I changed my shoes and went back. But I'd put on the other pair of mismatched shoes. Sometimes I can't think—the disease robs me of thought, and fills my mind with white static.

"My boss thought I was being stubborn and disrespectful. After that, things at work went downhill fast, and they forced me to leave. After all the paperwork was completed, I found out I was a few weeks' short on my time of employment with the railroad, and I missed out on my pension."

*

"White static." Chuck's words perfectly described Alzheimer's merciless march, not merely through the victim's brain, but through his or her life.

The sticky proteins collect, the neurons die. They will not be back. When the right neurons die, you lose crucial abilities, and white static covers all.

Chuck was taking his medications, hoping they would slow the disease's progress. He refused to shrink from new challenges. He confronted problems. He kept his brain working. He didn't withdraw from human contact, as had many of our relatives before him.

At the end of the day, Chuck and I were both tired. But I needed to ask him one more question. "You're the first of our family—the only one so far—to take the test to find out if you have the gene before you had any symptoms. What was that like?"

"I knew the odds, fifty-fifty. But, still, I was shocked to hear the words—to find out that I was unlucky, I had the gene," Chuck said.

"After being down about it, I promised myself I wouldn't give up. And my daughter—I promised her, too."

My flight left Portland on time the next day. We were six miles above the western landscape, too high to see the details of farms, barns, fences, and animals. But I could see the circles that told me where wells had been sunk into the aquifer, where center-pivot irrigation systems had been used to pump water out of the earth onto chemically fertilized, government-subsidized crops, in an area too dry and infertile to rely on natural climate and soil.

I tried to read, but I couldn't concentrate. I thought of the white static Chuck had described. My body tingled. I had so much to think about that I couldn't think about anything.

I wanted everything to fit: my experience in Oregon, my whole life to that point. The trouble was, nothing seemed to mesh. My grandson was about to get married; my son soon might be a grandfather, making me a great-grandfather. We had much to celebrate and look forward to. But I was reluctant to dwell on happiness. It didn't seem right in the context of the trip I'd just taken.

I had visited a cousin fighting a battle he would inevitably lose, as had his brother, his mother, his grandfather, and on and on. Yet I found myself hoping, praying for a miracle, something that might help him before it was too late.

And then I made a vow. I vowed I would run no more. I wouldn't lose contact with my cousin. Maybe I couldn't help him, but his courage had already helped me tremendously.

When I started writing this book, I stopped running. I began to sit still and listen. I listened to what Chuck told me, to what others told me, and, above all, to my own experience. I remembered what Chuck said about the white static robbing him of thought. I had changed the pace of my life, from the outer-directed life of doing and earning to a life of contemplation. I had chosen a life of contemplation when I became a minister, fifty years ago. But I wasn't ready then.

For years, I wrestled with fear about the family disease, afraid it might take my life away from me before I was ready to go. But now the disease had helped me find the life I have always wanted.

I looked out the window and saw a river and mountains, probably the eastern foothills of the Rockies. I reached in my briefcase and pulled out a book. Now I could read; I could concentrate; I could think. What a wonderful gift.

Chapter Fourteen

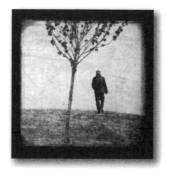

CHUCK'S GROUPIE

A *few months after I saw Chuck in Oregon, he and I sat together in a Senate hearing room in our nation's capital. Chuck had been invited to speak before the Senate. I wondered if this was the same room our Aunt Ester May had testified in twenty-five years earlier. After Chuck spoke, Dr. Rudolph Tanzi, one of the nation's best Alzheimer's researchers, spoke eloquently, if not humbly, about his role in searching for the genes, and now the cures for Alzheimer's.*

"*I am honored to be here this morning to address the Special Committee on Aging. I am a Professor of Neurology at Harvard Medical School and a geneticist at Massachusetts General Hospital. Twenty-five years ago, when I was a student at Harvard Medical School, I participated in the very first human genome mapping effort to locate a disease-causing gene. That gene was responsible for Huntington's disease. Shortly after, I focused my attention on mapping the genes for familial early onset Alzhiemer's disease, the type affecting Chuck." He turned and nodded respectfully toward my cousin.*

"In 1987, my lab discovered the first Alzheimer's gene and we identified two more in 1995, all three causing early onset Alzheimer's. I will summarize the tremendous amount we have learned about the causes of AD and the ongoing trials of new Alzheimer's drugs made possible by studies of these early onset AD genes.

"First, none of the discoveries or drug trials would be possible without the courageous involvement of patients, like Chuck. Second, few, if any, novel Alzheimer's drugs being developed by the pharmaceutical industry today would have been possible without the original seeds of creativity and basic biological and genetic discoveries that have come from academic research, primarily supported by federal and other non-profit funding for Alzheimer's research. Third, it generally takes about twenty years for basic research findings to reach the stage of clinical trials in patients. This is the case for the discovery of the first Alzheimer's genes in 1987, biological studies of those genes, and current clinical trials in 2008.

"While current Alzheimer's drugs only treat the symptoms offering minimal and temporary benefit to patients, several new Alzheimer's therapies currently in clinical trials are aimed at actually stopping the progression of the disease by curbing accumulation of toxic A-beta molecules in the brain. This can be achieved in three ways: one, limiting the production of A-beta; two, clearing A-beta out of the brain; and, three, neutralizing A-beta's toxic properties. Novel drugs of all three classes are currently in clinical trials, including a promising one that my lab helped develop over the last ten years.

"While I am optimistic about success, history dictates that the first drugs out of the gate are not always the best ones. We will clearly need to take many shots on goal; and, will most likely,

someday, be prescribing a cocktail of different drugs to effectively treat Alzheimer's.

"The most promising new drugs have been made possible from the knowledge gained from the studies of the gene defects causing early onset Alzheimer's. But these three genes along with one other for late onset account for only thirty percent of the inheritance of Alzheimer's disease. To find these, my lab at Massachusetts General Hospital is heading up the Alzheimer's Genome Project. A paper describing the first set of genes is currently under review at a major scientific journal, and we expect to announce several novel Alzheimer's genes this summer.

"So, while there is good reason to be optimistic, there is also a lot more work to do before we reach our goal. Scientists will need to work more closely than ever with clinicians, patients, the government, non-profits, and pharmaceutical companies to make this happen."[1]

T hree months after I saw Chuck in Oregon, I met up with him again in Washington, D.C. The Alzheimer's Association had invited him to participate in its 2008 Public Policy Forum, a platform for educating members and lobbying for funding from the U.S. legislature.

A week before the forum, Chuck wrote to me: "Big news. I've been invited to give testimony before the Senate Special Committee on Aging." It had been more than twenty-five years since Aunt Ester gave her testimony before Congress—the testimony that helped fund the Alzheimer's Disease Research Centers and led to the discovery of three early onset Alzheimer's genes, including the one that affects our family. It seemed that some mythical circle would be completed when Chuck, her nephew, spoke before the Senate.

---

[1] Notes of the author, May 14, 2008.

An hour after I arrived in Washington, I had lunch with Chuck and his daughter, Reba. Reba didn't know if she inherited the gene for early onset Alzheimer's from her dad; nor had she decided if she wanted to know. But she knew she wanted to have children. If she had the gene, she had that same fifty-fifty chance of passing it to her children. And Reba was already in her early thirties. Even if she had kids soon, they'd only be teenagers when she reached the average age of onset in our family. They'd be about the age Chuck was when he found his mother naked in the culvert.

The researchers in Seattle already had Reba's blood and had run the test, so the information was available if she decided she wanted to know. She'd need to have genetic counseling, like her father had, before obtaining the information.

When we got up from lunch, Reba went to the ladies' room, and I followed Chuck out. He was about to have his picture taken to accompany an article in the *Washington Post*. He walked with a languid stride, as if he had just taken off his barnyard overshoes for a trip into town. He looked a little disheveled, like a man just off the farm—or, perhaps, a man living with Alzheimer's. His sport coat had caught in the back of his pants. "Let's get this jacket out of your pants," I said. I left the rest to the photographer.

As we walked through the hotel lobby to meet the photographer, several people stopped Chuck, pumped his hand, and patted him on the back. Some of them were Alzheimer's Association staff people. But there were others, too, people he had met at the Public Policy Forum the year before, and people who had seen him on the video that I'd watched on *The New York Times* website. Chuck didn't know most of these people, but he greeted them with the grace and pleasure of a celebrity who hadn't yet tired of his fame.

After Reba rejoined us, she smoothed down Chuck's hair, and they got ready for their picture. The photographer wanted a picture of Chuck with Reba in the background, symbolizing the next generation.

*

The evening session, called the Public Policy Forum, was a cross between a fundamentalist revival meeting and a political convention. The head of each state's Alzheimer's Association gave a "state of the state" report.

After the state reports, various people with early stage Alzheimer's related their experiences following their diagnoses. One woman, evoking Hawthorne's protagonist Hester Prynne, said, "Once I was diagnosed with Alzheimer's, I felt I wore a big A on my forehead. People stopped talking to me, assuming I could not carry on a conversation."

Then Chuck stood up, wearing an Alzheimer's Association purple shirt bearing the words "Lend Your Voice." He said, with some fumbling and hesitation, "The medicines have helped me to where I am today. Of course, I'd trade to go back to a time when I didn't have Alzheimer's, but I have learned so much from having the disease and at times have a more intense joy than before I had it."

After breakfast the next morning, an Alzheimer's Association staffer whisked us by limo to the ABC affiliate in Washington where Chuck was scheduled for an interview to be aired the next day—the day of the Senate hearing. In front of the building, Chuck asked to be excused so he could have a cigarette.

Inside, Reba told me her dad felt smarter and more capable of answering questions after a smoke. I remembered some research that suggested nicotine helped short-term memory. But I wondered if Chuck should be left outside alone. What if he got confused about where we were, which doorway we'd entered? That kind of thing could happen to anyone. But my concern was unwarranted. In a few minutes, Chuck sauntered in, hyped up for another Alzheimer's celebrity moment.

I asked Chuck if he knew about the research that suggested nicotine helped short-term memory. He said, "Oh yes, that's why I smoke. If it helps rats, it should help me."

Reba and I watched the interview on a monitor. Chuck had brought the family picture he'd used so effectively in *The New York Times* video. When he started pointing to our relatives, I started to cry. I felt a mixture of pride at the way Chuck was dealing with his future and deep sadness for the family members who had died with Alzheimer's. I turned away from Reba so she wouldn't see my tears.

The next morning, we got our first glimpse of the *Washington Post* article, "Man With Alzheimer's Fights 'Family Disease.'" The picture of Chuck and Reba effectively portrayed the generational threat. The article, by staff writer Susan Levine, began: "When Chuck . . . takes his seat this morning before a U.S. Senate committee, he'll not lack for names or faces as he talks about the devastation that a disease called Alzheimer's has visited upon his family. His grandfather . . . a dozen aunts and uncles . . . his mother . . . a brother . . . plus every year, a growing list of cousins."[2]

🍃

Chuck had been told he would be the first to speak at the Senate hearing. But after we arrived, he was moved into the second group of speakers. The first group included Sandra Day O'Connor, the retired Supreme Court Justice, and Newt Gingrich, former Speaker of the House of Representatives.

The former Supreme Court Justice had been caring for her husband since 1990, when he received his Alzheimer's diagnosis. Newt Gingrich shared information about the Alzheimer's Study Group, which he co-chairs with former U.S. Senator Bob Kerrey. He explained that he first encountered the cruelty of Alzheimer's when he taught a Bible study class. "I watched with both frustration and sadness as the disease claimed one of my good friends," he said. Gingrich had many straightforward, well-thought-out suggestions about coordinating research and streamlining service delivery for the disease. Much to my surprise, Gingrich struck me as the best, most informed, and most powerful Alzheimer's advocate in America.

We'd been in the hearing room for nearly three hours when the second group of speakers, including Chuck, was called to the table. The room was

---

[2] *Washington Post*, Wednesday, May 14, 2008.

124

only half as full as it had been for O'Connor and Gingrich. Some of the senators had left. Most of those in the audience wore the purple ribbon bands of the Alzheimer's Association.

Before he slid into the chair behind the microphone, Chuck told me, "I can't see to read. This happens to me sometimes. That static thing. If I had gone first, I'd have been okay. If I could have had a cigarette, that would have helped, too."

"Just speak your heart," I said. "You were great yesterday without reading anything. You'll do fine."

Senator Gordon Smith of Oregon, the ranking member of the committee, introduced Chuck. Chuck started by saying he wouldn't follow the printed text word for word, but he didn't explain why. He showed the senators our family picture and explained that ten of the fourteen people in his mother's generation had early onset Alzheimer's.

He told them that the disease's symptoms had caught him by surprise, even though he knew he had the gene. Then he told the senators he wanted to live at home as long as possible. That was one of the points Gingrich emphasized: the need for supportive home services that would enable people to stay out of nursing homes for as long as possible. Chuck also listed his sources of income and told the senators, "I want you to know this disease is a very expensive thing to have. I have no money left at the end of the month."

Finally, Chuck told the senators he believed there are thousands of people who have undiagnosed early onset Alzheimer's. Doctors often don't recognize the disease in younger people, and those with symptoms often are afraid or ashamed to talk about them. "If my mother's generation had only talked about what was happening to them in the 1960s, we would have more done today," he said.

The next speaker, Suzanne Carbone, was a librarian and a caregiver for her husband, Bob. Bob is an identical twin, but his twin brother has no symptoms. Researchers have yet to solve this mystery. She was followed by Rudolph Tanzi, professor of neurology and neuroscience at Harvard University and director of the Genetics and Aging Unit of Massachusetts General Hospital.

Dr. Tanzi has been in the forefront of the research on Alzheimer's disease since the early 1980s. He first worked on tracing the gene for Huntington's disease, and then, using that same technique, made significant contributions to the discovery of all three early onset Alzheimer's genes: APP on chromosome 21, PS1 on chromosome 14, and PS2, the Volga German gene, our gene, on chromosome 1. In addition to his academic and research work, Dr. Tanzi "is a principal scientific founder of Prana Biotechnology, Ltd.; Geneplex, Inc.; and Neurogenetics, Inc. Dr. Tanzi has equity in all three companies as well as the publicly traded companies Elan Pharmaceuticals and Bristol-Myers Squibb."[3]

Now it was twenty-five years since Aunt Ester testified before Congress, twenty-three years after the Alzheimer's Disease Research Centers were funded across the nation, and thirteen years after the gene that affects our family had been found. Yet not much had changed since the day in August, 1995, I picked up *The New York Times* and learned that scientists had isolated our gene. Would Dr. Tanzi—perhaps the nation's best Alzheimer's researcher—reveal something new?

I harbored muted hopes that we'd hear some as yet unrevealed good news.

*

In 2000, a reporter for the *New York Times* asked Dr. Tanzi, "How close are we to an effective treatment for Alzheimer's disease?" The doctor replied, "I wouldn't be surprised if five years from now we have a pretty effective drug that can slow the disease down enough so that it will be preventable in those at risk, and significantly slow down the deterioration of people who already have it." He added, "If you compare Alzheimer's to heart disease where cholesterol levels must be lowered, we now have our own cholesterol equivalent,

---

[3] Tanzi, Rudolph E., & Parson, Ann B., *Decoding Darkness:The Search for the Genetic Causes of Alzheimer's Disease*, Perseus Publishing: New York, 2000, credits page.

which we call the beta amyloid. The name of the game in Alzheimer's therapy is lowering the accumulation of beta amyloid in the brain."[4]

But now eight years later, Dr. Tanzi, speaking to the Senate Select Committee on Aging, said, "Alzheimer's drugs only treat the symptoms, offering minimal and only temporary benefit to patients."

Dr. Tanzi repeatedly emphasized that research conducted on early onset families had provided crucial new information about the disease. "These are pioneering days, and the future is bright," he said. "Scientists will need to work more closely than ever with clinicians, patients, the government, nonprofits, and pharmaceutical companies to ensure further progress."

He added that the potential therapies are still in clinical trials. Most of them aim to stop the progression of the disease by curbing the accumulation of beta amyloid in the brain, the assumed culprit in Alzheimer's. "While I am optimistic about the success of these trials, history dictates that the first drugs out of the gate are not always the best ones," he admitted.

Changing metaphors from horse racing to hockey, he added, "We will clearly need to take many shots on goal to cure this disease; and, will most likely, someday, be prescribing a cocktail of different drugs to effectively treat Alzheimer's."

Those were the three most chilling words of the day: "most likely, someday." I'd hoped for better news for Chuck's sake, and for Reba's sake, and for my nieces and nephews' sake, and for the sake of all my relatives who were facing the age of onset. But especially for Chuck. Because he still had enough mind power left that even if a drug didn't reverse the disease — if it merely stopped its progress — he could still live a long, productive life.

But, it seemed Dr. Tanzi's easy optimism at the turn of the new millennium had ceded to the reality of a longer struggle. Despite the discovery of our gene and two other early onset genes, and a fourth gene associated with late onset Alzheimer's, not much had changed.

---

[4]*The New York Times*, December 5, 2000.

After the hearing, I approached Dr. Tanzi. I introduced myself and told him my family was one of the families involved in the Volga German research conducted by his friend Gerard Schellenberg and Dr. Bird and his associates in Seattle. Dr. Tanzi interrupted me and said, "I found that gene, you know."

I must have looked surprised, because he exclaimed, "I did!" But I wasn't surprised to hear he'd found the gene; I knew there had been intense competition between several labs. I was surprised he felt the need to claim sole credit. He had said in his book that he had called Schellenberg in Seattle and told him about the homolog (to the gene on chromosome 14) on chromosome 1 because he knew that being a good colleague instead of a rival was important for the research to progress. He could have looked for the gene on chromosome 1 himself because he had access to a frozen Volga German brain stored in the freezer at Mass General. With the knowledge of the homolog, he might have beaten Schellenberg and Bird out and found the gene despite the fact they'd been sifting the DNA of the Volga Germans for almost ten years.

"I'm wondering if I could talk to you," I said. "I'm working on a book about the impact of the disease on our family."

Again, he cut me short. "Here's how you should contact me," he said. He turned to a big man behind his right shoulder and told him, "Give him your card."

The man reached around Dr. Tanzi and handed me his card. FRANCIS, EDWARD, & CRONIN, INC., Strategic, Nonprofit, & Governmental Affairs Management. The big man was a consultant, a manager—exactly the kind of companion Dr. Tanzi needed. The doctor had many details to keep straight, and a tight schedule to meet. Besides that, he might be sitting on the edge of a fortune if the drug trials work out. There was so much to gain and so much to lose. It was important to have the right man at his side.

Suddenly I felt guilty for wanting to talk to Dr. Tanzi. Who was I to waste a great man's time, one of the best scientists in the country? I couldn't even think of anything I wanted to ask him. Maybe I had selfishly hoped for a publicity blurb for this book, from the famous researcher who had helped find our defective gene, who has done so much to help our family and give us hope.

Then I got angry. As Dr. Tanzi followed the big man out of the hearing room of the U.S. Senate, I wanted to shout, "That was our blood you looked at under the microscope! That frozen brain you had in the freezer at Mass General might have been the brain of the uncle I loved, who came home safe from the war and married a local beauty. Just because we were research subjects doesn't mean. . . ."

Then I didn't know what it didn't mean. . . I just felt like I wanted to cry.

I looked over my shoulder and saw Chuck coming toward me. He put his hand on my shoulder. "How did I do?" he asked.

I turned to look him in the eye, taking a few seconds to compose myself. "You were great," I said. "You were better off not reading. You kept their attention by looking at them and just saying what was on your mind."

"Thanks," he said. "I know I fumbled a little bit."

"No, you did great!" I repeated.

"Did you have a good talk with Dr. Tanzi?" Chuck asked.

"No, no I didn't," I answered. "I didn't like it at all. But I like following you around, being your groupie."

"Man, I have to say, you sure are an ugly groupie."

Before I could reply, Chuck punched my shoulder with a solid right hook. That's the way we panhandle men show affection.

Chapter Fifteen

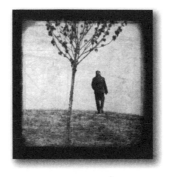

THE SCIENCE PROJECT

W*illiam Klunk, M.D., Ph.D.,
professor of psychiatry and neurology, and Chester Mathis, Ph.D.,
professor of radiology and pharmaceutical sciences, both from the
University of Pittsburgh, ran laboratory experiments to find a
compound that would safely pass through the blood-brain barrier
and bind to the beta amyloid proteins in the brain that make up
the plaques, the distinguishing markers of Alzheimer's disease.
After nearly ten years of experiments, they succeeded with the
Pittsburgh Compound (PiB).*

*Because the compound binds to the proteins then clears out
of the brain, they found they could inject it with a low dose of
radioactivity and use a PET scan to photograph the brain revealing
the precise arrangement of plaques. To prove the accuracy of this
procedure, they scanned the brains of some volunteers who had been
diagnosed with Alzheimer's. At their death, their brains were studied*

in autopsy. The scientists demonstrated that the pictures accurately revealed the location and extent of the toxic proteins in the brains of the volunteers. For the first time, a definitive diagnosis of Alzheimer's became possible before death and autopsy.

But diagnosis is, perhaps, the least of the uses of PiB. As already noted, it will be used in the DIAN study to reveal the development of Alzheimer's before symptoms even occur. The scientists hope this will lead to treatments that can stop the progress of the disease before it damages the brain.

Since other substances are being tested that have shown the possibility of actually dissolving the harmful proteins of Alzheimer's disease, PiB might be used in the future as a conductor of another substance that would reverse existing symptoms.

F our months after my trip to Washington with Chuck and Reba, I drove from New York to Pittsburgh to meet up with Chuck and his ex-wife, Marianne. Although they had separated and divorced a few years ago, they were back together, living in the same house they lived in when they were married.

After I checked in to my hotel, I sat down in the lobby to wait for them. My cell phone rang. Checking the readout, I saw it was my Aunt Marie in Oklahoma. This couldn't be good news. My aunt had said during our visit with Anne in the nursing home, "I wish the good Lord would take her," and I supposed her wish had come true.

When I answered the call, it was not my aunt but her grandson, Anne's younger son. "Gary," he said, "Granny asked me to call and tell you that Uncle Karl passed away." My mind skittered. I almost said, "I thought it was probably your mother who died." But I avoided saying anything just long enough to avoid saying the wrong thing.

"Granny's hoping you'll be able to come to the funeral," he said.

"Can I talk to her for a moment?" I asked.

"She just cries," he said. "She can't talk."

"Tell her I'll be there," I said. "Tell her I'll be there, and tell her I love her."

My cousin Karl was the younger child of Uncle Otto and Aunt Marie. The last time I saw him, Karl could only speak a word or two before his speech broke into babble, but he recognized me and said "Gary" and "cousin." A few months after I saw him, his wife had to place him in an Alzheimer's care facility. When she tried to help him to bed, he thought she was a stranger and summoned enough language to scream one sentence: "Get the hell out of my house." When she tried to calm him, he hit her and blackened her eye; then he swung at their son when he came to help. But despite his deteriorating condition, he didn't seem to be in danger of dying. I wondered what had happened.

But at that moment, I had to concentrate on why I was in Pittsburgh: to support Chuck while the Pittsburgh Compound (PiB) was tested on him, and to find out what the Pittsburgh Compound was all about.

To test PiB, researchers needed people in the early stages of Alzheimer's disease. Chuck volunteered because he wanted to help advance the research, which might lead to better treatments and, in the most optimistic view, possibly reverse the effects of the disease. Chuck wants the next generation— including his daughter and others in our family who may have inherited the gene—to have more options. That mission keeps him going.

He also harbors the long-shot hope that he might stumble into a miraculous cure that will reverse his own symptoms before it's too late. He knows he doesn't have much time left.

The study on PiB isn't the only research in which Chuck participates. He and his older brother, Darin, whose symptoms are much more advanced than Chuck's, are both receiving Elan infusions, the Alzheimer's vaccine that produces antibodies to the beta amyloid proteins (A-beta) that accumulate in the brains of Alzheimer's sufferers. The vaccine's effectiveness has been demonstrated on rodents, and human trials are now entering their second phase. The trials were suspended in 2002 when thirteen of the 300 participants developed brain inflammation; three of them died. Researchers have developed a safer vaccine for the new phase.

The Elan study is blind. No one knows who gets the vaccine and who gets the placebo. Chuck recently reported some improvement in Darin's math ability. Before the study, Chuck's brother "could not even figure out one plus one." But now he could recognize numbers and solve some simple math problems.

Chuck hasn't noticed any dramatic improvement in his own brain function, although he senses the disease is advancing more slowly than it does in many other Alzheimer's sufferers. Of course, Chuck has no way of knowing if he's receiving the vaccine or a placebo. He can only hope it's the former.

The laboratory at the University of Pittsburgh spent ten years developing the Pittsburgh Compound. The compound, which contains a low dose of radioactivity, is attracted to and adheres to the A-beta proteins that accumulate in the brains of people with Alzheimer's. The radioactive material shows up on the PET scans so researchers can photograph the amyloid protein deposits and precisely measure changes from test to test. Researchers have compared these photographs to the brains of people who died of Alzheimer's and confirmed the photos' accuracy.

To this point in time, scientists have obtained a definitive diagnosis of Alzheimer's by dissection after death, just as Dr. Alzheimer did with the brain of Frau Auguste D when he first discovered the plaques and tangles more than a hundred years ago. Besides dissection, the most effective way to diagnose the disease has been through tests and interviews. The most skilled diagnostic clinics are more than ninety percent accurate in identifying Alzheimer's in the early stages. But diagnosis can only occur after symptoms occur; many experts agree that effective treatment should begin *before* symptoms occur. That's another reason the Pittsburgh Compound is so important: it may enable scientists to photograph and analyze accumulated plaque before patients start to experience symptoms. Theoretically, Alzheimer's screening could become part of an annual physical examination after a certain age, like screening for breast or prostate cancer. Those who are genetically at risk might receive even earlier screening.

PiB may also help determine which drugs are effective on Alzheimer's patients. Currently, measuring drugs' effectiveness is a long process. After a patient experiences symptoms, doctors prescribe and administer drugs; they then use tests and interviews to measure any change in the patient's conditions. Since PiB adheres to the A-beta proteins but clears out of normal tissue quickly, doctors can use scans and photos to measure the drugs' effects on the amount of A-beta proteins in the brain.

The most improbable but exciting use for PiB might be as a conductor for other compounds that might dissolve A-beta proteins and reverse the disease. The brain is protected by an intricate system called the blood/brain barrier, which prevents most substances from entering the brain. Since PiB can penetrate this barrier, it might be an ideal transportation system for a plaque-dissolving compound.

But researchers still have major challenges ahead. They've yet to prove that the A-beta proteins cause Alzheimer's. Some scientists believe the proteins are a *result* of the disease, not the cause. Chuck hopes he can help them learn the truth.

*

Chuck and Marianne arrived at the hotel and went to their room to get settled. Dr. Klunk would pick us up later and take us to dinner. While Chuck and Marianne were in their room, I thought about how I should tell them that our cousin Karl had died. I'd just as soon not bring it up at all. Karl was only three years older than Chuck. A chill goes through my body every time I hear of another Alzheimer's death in our family. I can't imagine what the news does to Chuck and Marianne, since Chuck knows he's on the same path. But it would be awkward if they found out I knew Karl had died and hadn't told them.

When we met in the lobby before dinner, I told them. "Aunt Marie called a few hours ago to tell me Karl died." Chuck didn't seem surprised. I told him the family had set up a website on which we could post our thoughts and condolences. Chuck said he would do so. "I know it will mean a lot coming from you," I said.

Dr. Klunk arrived and greeted Chuck and Marianne. They introduced me to him. In April, Dr. Klunk and two colleagues had been awarded the Potamkin Prize, referred to as the "Nobel Prize for Neurology," given to scientists who make significant contributions to understanding and treatment of Alzheimer's disease and related dementias.

At dinner, Dr. Klunk asked Chuck how he'd been doing since the last time they'd seen each other, a couple of years ago. Chuck told him he'd attended the Alzheimer's Association Public Policy Forum in Washington and had testified before the Senate Special Committee On Aging, and he told Dr. Klunk how he spent his time when he was at home.

Dr. Klunk told Chuck, "You seem to be holding your own. You seem good." I thought of Chuck outside the hotel smoking a cigarette. He had inhaled his favorite memory enhancer minutes before Dr. Klunk arrived.

Chuck looked pleased and said, "I think the cocktail of medications I'm on is helping." As Chuck talked to Dr. Klunk, a frown lingered on Marianne's face. After Chuck spoke, it was Marianne's turn. Her voice was so soft and the restaurant so noisy I heard only a few words, but I heard enough to understand that she offered a more sobering opinion. Maybe there were some worrisome changes. Chuck poked his food with a fork.

Back at the hotel, I ordered single-malt scotches for Chuck and me, and then we got on the website that our cousin Karl's wife and sons had set up. In his message Chuck said he was sorry he couldn't be at Karl's funeral, and noted that at these times when the family should gather to support one another, he was very aware how far the family had scattered. As he was pecking out his condolences, he told me he thought Alzheimer's disease had been a factor in how far the family had dispersed. I said I couldn't agree more.

The next morning, the three of us, led by a social worker from the research lab, trudged up cardiac hill, as the incline has always been called. When we reached the lab that conducts the PET scans, the researchers led Chuck away for a fitting. The last time Chuck was scanned, lab workers had warmed a plastic mask and then molded it to his face. Now they wanted to make sure his mask still fit. When Chuck returned, the nurse had the mask in her hand. I noticed several buckles fastened to the mask. The nurse explained that lab workers strap Chuck's head down so he couldn't move even a fraction of an inch during the two-hour scan. Hearing this, I felt so panicked and dizzy I thought I might pass out.

After the scan, Chuck was disoriented, but he felt better when he had some lunch. The nurse gave Chuck some chocolate, explaining that it helps increase brain activity.

There was one more thirty-minute scan to come. Some scientists have theorized that brains can create new learning pathways to bypass diseased sections. The second scan would determine whether there was any new neuronal activity in Chuck's brain.

I hadn't heard from Aunt Marie or her grandson, so while Chuck was having his second scan, I called Karl's wife to offer my condolences and to get the funeral details. I told her Karl had seemed physically healthy the last time I saw him. She said he'd gone downhill after he went into the nursing home. "It was heartbreaking," she said, but she couldn't keep him at home anymore. About ten days ago, he had stopped eating and drinking. Even when she brought his favorite ice cream, he kept his teeth clenched. After a few days of refusing all intake, he got a fever. When his mother visited him, he was conscious and recognized her. But soon after seeing her, he went into a coma, and he died within a few hours. His widow added, "This had to be what he wanted. I have no other explanation."

There I was in Pittsburgh with my cousin Chuck, who was showing enormous courage and giving hope to the next generation and those to follow — and now came news of another kind of courage, the grit that enabled Karl to use his last measure of mental acuity to shorten his life, to spare his family what his sister and her sons were going through and what he had gone through with his own dad.

Karl's death was very hard for my Aunt Marie to bear, but it would have been even harder for her to bear the drawn-out confinement of her son in a long-term care facility. She already had that experience with her daughter.

After Chuck's second scan, the social worker led us back down cardiac hill to the hotel. We rested for an hour then met in the lobby for a walk to the Phipps Conservatory, a garden near Schenley Park, at the edge of the university campus. The conservatory was the site of the annual Easter flower show. My first wife and our children had walked to the conservatory every Easter after church to see the flowers. As Chuck, Marianne, and I approached the building, I could almost see my young daughter in a new dress with crinolines, and the two boys, almost like twins, walking ahead of us with their hands in their pockets, pretending to be older than they were. I felt tears along the rims of my eyelids. I wanted to pull Chuck close, tell him how much I admired him and loved him for what he was doing for our family and many others unknown to me. I asked Chuck and Marianne to pose in front of a large exotic plant. I snapped a photo. Instead of the extraordinary people they are, they looked like just an ordinary couple doing some sight seeing.

After we had dinner together, we returned to the hotel, and Chuck and Marianne went to their room. I had said good-bye to my cousin and his wife. Soon I would see my beautiful Aunt Marie, who cries more than she talks.

Chapter Sixteen

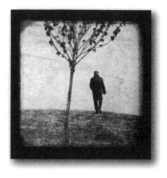

LAST MAN STANDING

 F *orty-five years ago when my Aunt*
Ester May carted my Uncle George from doctor to doctor to find
out what was wrong with him, only one had the idea it was
Alzheimer's disease. Thirty years ago, the University of Colorado
sent my family mimeographed letters announcing information
meetings about Alzheimer's, but the information available could
be summarized in a brief sentence: There's not much to report.

The explosion of knowledge, awareness, and research about
Alzheimer's is a phenomenon that could be called miraculous.
And, now we have the internet, a little more powerful than the
mimeograph used to circulate the announcements sent out by the
University of Colorado.

Within five minutes on the internet, I found the following
articles available for anyone to read: Closing In On Origins Of
Main Ingredient Of Alzheimer's Plaques; Naturally Occurring

Enzyme Can Break Down Key Part of Alzheimer's Plaques; Mediterranean Diet May Help Alzheimer's; Epilepsy Drug Could Prevent and Treat Alzheimer's; Depression is a Risk Factor Rather Than Early Sign of Alzheimer's Disease; University Of Kentucky Researcher Uncovers Clues To Alzheimer's Disease; How Big Is Your Brain? Its Size May Protect You From Memory Loss; UC Davis Study Shows Estrogen Protects Brain Cells And Reduces Risk of Developing Alzheimer's Disease; Learning Slows Physical Progression Of Alzheimer's Disease; Alzheimer's Disease Risk Factors May Be Gender-Specific; Diabetes Link To Alzheimer's Disease Explained; Higher Folate Levels Linked To Reduced Risk For Alzheimer's Disease; Optical Scientists, Psychiatrists Develop Minimally Invasive Eye Test For Alzheimer's; Research Links Fast Food To Alzheimer's; A Genetic GPS For Earlier Diagnosis; Another Puzzle-Piece Towards a Genetic Cure; Prana's Progress Inhibits Alzheimer's Damage; Reveral of Alzheimer's Symptoms Within Minutes Reported In New Study; Progress on the Oklahoma City Vaccination; Epix Trial Improved Alz Scores in Just Two Weeks; FDA-approved Gammagard Increases Antibodies That Clear Alzheimer's; Grant Awarded For Drug That Fights Alzheimer's On Multiple Fronts; Oxidative Stress—An Emerging Approach to Fighting Alzheimer's; New Alzheimer's Therapy Brings Hope; A Daily Cup of Coffee May Halt Alzheimer's.

This list of articles is only a fraction of what's available. The list can get trite and overwhelming, and may produce a bit of skepticism in any reasonable reader. But, the study of Alzheimer's disease and the effort and money being spent on the development of treatments to attack the disease from every possible angle is providing us all with hope, and it is keeping a lot of scientists employed.

I arrived at the Chisholm Creek Baptist Church in time to speak to and hug my Aunt Marie before everyone shuffled into the sanctuary for her son's memorial service.

I sat with Aunt Marie's grandson, his wife, his stepson, and his new baby boy. He is my cousin Anne's younger son who called me to tell me about Karl's death. He is the same age as my youngest son, Jesse; the two of them used to play together when we visited my mother and Aunt Marie in Oklahoma.

Anne's older son wasn't at his uncle's funeral. After he left Oklahoma, he'd lived in Japan, and he'd recently hopped over to Australia. He is ten years from the usual age of onset for the disease. He is married and also has a new baby boy. I wonder if he thinks he has escaped the disease by skipping from continent to continent. Doesn't he realize that his fate was sealed when his parents conceived him?

Homespun country music came over the speaker system. Karl loved country music. There was no coffin because Karl wished to be cremated. Cremation is an unusual way to dispose of a dead body in Oklahoma where there's plenty of space for cemeteries and graves, and where many fundamentalist Christians believe in the resurrection of the body and so tend to leave the body whole. Even my mother, with her highly practical views, refused to allow an autopsy on my father because she wanted to bury him intact. She said he had suffered enough humiliation during his lifetime. So none of his brain tissue was extracted for the research that began after his death.

Aunt Marie faced the same issue when Uncle Otto finally died. But his body was a mere shell of what it had been, and his brain hadn't been conscious for years, so she allowed science to have its way. When her son expressed his wish to be cremated, I knew she would respect his wishes.

The printed program gave the date Karl "entered life" (his birth date) and the date he "entered eternal life" (the date he died). A reader recited Psalm 23, "The Lord is my shepherd, I shall not want," followed by John 14,

"In my father's house are many mansions. If it were not so, I would have told you." Then we sang a hymn:

I come to the garden alone, while the dew is still on the roses,
And the voice I hear, falling on my ear, the Son of God discloses.
And He walks with me and He talks with me, and He tells me I
am His own.
And the joy we share as we tarry there, none other has ever
known.

A screen unrolled in front of the baptistery. Projectors came on, and pictures of Karl and his family appeared on the screen, two or three at the same time, fading in, fading out: Karl and his wife, his children, and his grandchildren; Karl when he was small, with his parents, Otto and Marie, and his sister, Anne.

Then the pastor preached. He told us he had gone to the nursing home to visit Karl. He spoke to Karl about the merciful Christ, the forgiving God. He asked Karl if it would be okay if he prayed, and Karl seemed to give his mute consent. The pastor prayed, "God be merciful to me, a sinner." He repeated the prayer several times, tapping Karl's knee each time, and then asked Karl if he understood. "Tap if you want to pray," the pastor said to Karl. Karl raised his fingers and tapped his leg, and the pastor prayed, "God be merciful to me, a sinner."

The pastor closed the service by asking everyone to bow their heads and close their eyes. "Raise your hand if you will pray this prayer," he said. "Raise your hand," he pleaded. He repeated the prayer: "God be merciful unto me, a sinner. God be merciful unto me, a sinner."

In spite of my skeptic's mind, my heart felt comforted by this service because I believed Karl was comforted by the pastor's call at the nursing home. It may have been that visit that helped Karl muster the strength and mental awareness to refuse food and drink and speed his trip into eternity. I wished Karl "God speed" as the pastor said, "Amen."

The family gathered in the church fellowship hall for meat, scalloped potatoes, casseroles, Jell-O salads, and pumpkin pie. Much has changed in funerals since I was a minister—nowadays there's country music and multi-media—but the menu remains the same.

I sat with my dear aunt, other relatives, and people from home I hadn't seen for many years, and we chatted and ate until our bellies were as full as our souls. Before Aunt Marie was whisked away by her sister, she gave me a big, teary hug and thanked me "for coming all this way."

When I flew back to Pittsburgh to pick up my car and drive home, I fell into a contemplative state, just as I'd done after visiting Chuck in Oregon. Once again, I felt alone, although I was squeezed into an airplane seat amid dozens of others. In my loneliness, I lapsed into a memory from childhood.

When the bell rings for recess, we go outside to lay out the course for our favorite game, Fox and Geese. Beyond the swings and the merry-go-round, snow gleams level and undisturbed on the softball field. Ben and Bryant, the oldest kids in school, order everyone else to stay back and not make any tracks while they make the first pass. Then the rest of us follow, carefully tramping down the snow so the edges are sharp and we can tell exactly when someone goes out of bounds. The course is laid out in the shape of a freshly sliced pie, with paths that lead to the center, or the goose pen—a safe haven where the geese can temporarily avoid being caught by the fox. To kill a goose and eliminate it from the game, the fox must touch it with both hands. The last goose alive becomes the fox for the next game. I want to be the fox. I want to be sly, instinctive, cunning.

Several boys, including me, start arguing about who gets to be the fox. But Ben insists it should be him, since he's the oldest. The rest of us give in.

Ben chases the younger kids first, so they won't be in the way when the *real* chasing begins. He makes the kids run, lagging just behind them so they'll be frightened for a few seconds. That's the point. If you're not afraid of being caught and killed, you're not really playing the game.

Soon there are only five geese alive, including my sister and me. My sister heads to the goose pen to rest. I join her.

"Ben likes you," I say. "He's not even trying to catch you." In an instant, she's angry—whether at Ben or me I'm not sure. She leaves the goose pen. Ben starts after her, but it's a ruse; when I step out behind them, he reverses, and before I can turn and run, he puts both hands on my head and says, "You're dead, goose." He laughs raucously.

At first I don't feel anything, but as I walk off the course to join the other dead geese, I get mad. I walk to the merry-go-round, knock some snow off the seat, sit down, and give it a kick. When I look back, Ben has caught another boy. Ben wants to save my sister until last—no, next to last. If she's last, he won't get to touch her. And that's the whole point of the game for him.

Ben catches another boy. Now there are only two geese left. Ben starts after my sister, who doesn't run. "I don't want to be the fox," she says.

"You have to run," he says.

"I'm not running. You may as well get it over with." My sister walks toward Ben, but he backs up. She speeds up; so does he. Someone yells, "The goose is chasing the fox!"

Then my sister stops running. "I'm going in," she says. She turns her back on Ben and starts heading toward the schoolhouse. She cuts through the unmarked snow in the middle of the circle, spoiling the boundaries of the course. Ben comes up behind her and knocks her down. He drops on top of her, pins her arms. My sister screams, "Get off me!!" Some of the smaller kids run toward the schoolhouse.

Ben lets her hands go. She flails at him, trying to fight him off, but he ignores her gloved fists, and puts his hands first on her thighs, then her belly, and then higher and higher until they reach her breasts. "You're dead, goose," he says. "You are damned dead." He closes his fists, crumpling the fabric of her coat.

Before I realize it, I'm running toward him. Ben turns and starts to rise. His face is in line with my chest. I have my arms in front of me, elbows out, like a fullback about to lay a block. With the momentum of my speed, my forearm catches him flush on the nose. He falls backward, and blood gushes onto the snow. My sister gets to her feet and runs.

I know Ben's brothers are on their way to help him. Someone yells "Last man standing, last man standing. Come on, come on, last man standing." Ben gets up and staggers toward the schoolhouse, bending over so his nose won't bleed on him. The girls and a few of the boys head inside too. The others crowd into the Fox and Goose circle I'm standing in.

Last Man Standing is a game with just one rule: if you're down, you're out. I start to cry. I don't care if they think I'm a baby. Two boys, Jackie and Buddy, attack me straight on, with no strategy between them. I step aside and trip the overweight Buddy; before Jackie regains his balance, I hit him on the side of the head. He goes down. One by one, the others come after me: Bryant, J.D., Ronnie Patee, Kenny Ritterbush. I won't go down. I won't let my feet be taken out from under me. I will stand. I will be the last man standing.

And I am.

The bell rings, and I'm alone in the middle of the trampled, obliterated circle. When you are the last man standing, you are truly alone.

🍂

Back in Pittsburgh, I walked toward my car in the airport parking lot. I was glad I had a ten-hour drive back to East Hampton ahead of me. I needed some time to ponder why I felt both so lucky and so alone after being with Chuck and Marianne and Aunt Marie, and all the others.

🍂

Less than two months after returning from meeting up with Chuck in Pittsburgh, then attending Karl's funeral in Oklahoma, in my email was a note from another cousin's daughter in Arizona, a tall, slender woman in her thirties with a darling little daughter. My cousin had died. He was the older son of my Uncle George and my Aunt Ester May. This cousin had been a minister of youth and music in the church we both grew up in; he was musically talented, ebullient.

> Hello there, well, after his diagnosis with genetic, early onset Alzheimer's 8 1/2 years ago, my Dad is dancing and leading the choir and cracking jokes and working with the youth with his Savior in HEAVEN!!! I am so excited that he is finally relieved of his earthly body and brain!! I know that he and the rest of the Reiswig family members, including his dad, who suffered through this disease, are all comparing their "new" brains ☺.
>
> (My daughter) and I . . . went with my Mom to the nursing home at 10 am. When we got there my Dad was breathing heavily and loudly. It was very disconcerting. It made ME uncomfortable just listening to it. After a couple of hours, the breathing became less labored and quieter. A friend of my Mom and Dad's was there at 11am and another came at 2 pm. She left a few hours later and yet another friend came at 6 pm. All this time (my little daughter) was awesome!!! She walked around and chatted with the old folks (my dad was the youngest resident at 61 years of age . . . all the rest are in their 80's). They just loved her☺. I surprised myself at being able to sit and do nothing for 11 hours . . . don't know when the last time was that I did that. It felt good to be there with my Mom and just know that I was with my dad.
>
> So, his color continued to change and his breathing became more rapid for several hours. Then around 9 pm-ish his breathing became more shallow. It continued to slow down . . . my Mom was laying on the bed with my Dad just holding him. I was holding Alice and saw my dad take his last breath. WOW!!! I am so glad that I was able to be there and that my mom was holding her honey of 40 years when he went home to be with Jesus.
>
> We left around 11 pm just before the research institute came to pick up my Dad. Years ago, he arranged for his body/brain to be

donated to research. The Reiswig family has been under the microscope so to speak for a long time due to the uniqueness and prevalence of Alzheimer's in our family genetics. Who knows? Maybe my Dad's brain will be the key that unlocks this horrible disease and frees up the rest of his family ☺.

We are planning a memorial service for Saturday. It will be at Christ's Church of the Valley. . . . We are sad to lose our Dad but so excited that he is FREE AT LAST!!!

Thank you all for your prayers and support throughout the years. I love you all.

By HIS Grace,

(names omitted by author)

Chapter Seventeen

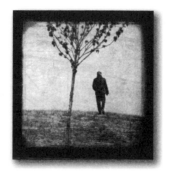

ODESSA INTERSECTION

I*n July, 2009, it was announced that Johnson & Johnson, the American pharmaceutical company, had agreed to pay the Irish biotechnology company, Elan, one billion dollars for what amounts to 18.4 percent of the company, despite the fact that Elan reported a loss of 112 million dollars in the first quarter of 2009.*

Johnson & Johnson will set up a company to continue Elan's partnership with Wyeth, one of the world's largest research-driven pharmaceutical and health care products companies. That alliance has been working on an Alzheimer's Immunotherapy Program (AIP), the one that my cousins Chuck and Darin partici-pate in. In addition to the one billion dollar investment in the company, Johnson & Johnson will invest a half billion into contin-uing the research and development of AIP, including work with bapineuzumab, a drug that shows great promise for slowing the progression of Alzheimer's disease. This drug is now moving into phase three clinical trials. As part of the deal, Elan will retain fifty percent of the production and profit of the new company.

It is exciting that a "for profit" company sees such potential in Alzheimer's treatments. Without their investment hope would hardly exist. But everyone concerned must ask this questions: Can a corporation driven by the profit motive in a game with such high stakes be scrupulously honest and altruistic? Every citizen, scientist, and elected official must be alert while wishing good luck and God speed to those who must make a profit to survive.

It's five o'clock in the morning. I can't sleep. I feel jittery, afraid. More than seventy years ago, my grandmother died when my granddad drove his truck onto the railroad crossing near Huntoon, Texas. Yesterday, I received a note from my nephew's wife telling me he had been in an accident at an intersection in Odessa, Texas. He received a ticket for a traffic violation; he was saved from serious injury by seatbelts and airbags. Had my nephew's wife been in the truck, she might have died. "The other guy was going too fast—hit him broadside," she told me.

My nephew is the oldest member of the next generation in line for Presenilin 2, the early onset Alzheimer's gene that runs in our family. His dad and his mom, my sister, took over the farm when my father's Alzheimer's advanced so far he could no longer operate it. My nephew was in partnership on the farm with his parents for more than a decade before he decided to get a job with steady pay and health insurance.

I'd spoken to my nephew's wife shortly before his accident in Odessa. She told me she'd noticed some changes in his behavior. He'd been a capable mechanic and repairman, as all farmers must be. She said, "Now, when I ask him to fix something around the house, he spends a lot of time looking for misplaced tools. I go out to the shop to see what's taking him so long. He tells me he's looking for a screwdriver. I pick one up off the bench. 'This one?' I ask. He's mystified that I've been able to find it so easily. He can look right at something, but it doesn't make it through to his brain." Then she softened her complaint. "I can't be too hard on him," she said. "I do the same thing. I'll put down a flour sifter and two minutes later I can't find it. But eventually I get the cake baked."

She paused and then said, "You spent some time with him on that trip to the reunion. What do you think?" Of course, I knew why she was asking. She knows I've seen Alzheimer's in my grandfather, my father and his generation, and my generation, including my brother and my sister.

I told her I didn't know if her husband was getting Alzheimer's, but I suggested that they go to an Alzheimer's clinic and get an evaluation. Even if everything seemed fine now, they could refer to that baseline evaluation if he showed symptoms in the future. But she said she and her husband didn't want any testing, especially genetic testing. They were afraid that if his employer found out about the family's genetic background, my nephew might lose his job and the family's insurance.

But my nephew needs an evaluation that might enable him to take drugs such as Namenda, Razadyne, and Aricept—a cocktail like the one my cousin, Chuck, takes in hopes of slowing down the disease. If my nephew was in the early phases of the disease, medications might delay more severe symptoms and help keep him employed longer. In addition, he'd be in the Alzheimer's network when new drugs became available, so he could get them more quickly. The earlier treatment begins, the more effective it is.

*

The Alzheimer's Association has a list of ten warning signs of Alzheimer's disease: *memory loss, difficulty performing familiar tasks, problems with language, disorientation to time and place, poor or decreased judgment, problems with abstract thinking, misplacing things, changes in mood or behavior, changes in personality, loss of initiative.*

151

A perfectly healthy person can exhibit any or all of these symptoms at one time or another. When diagnosing Alzheimer's, doctors look for the *degree* and *frequency* of these symptoms.

When my nephew and I were on our trip to the panhandle for a family reunion, he had some trouble remembering names. Several times I supplied the names of people we both knew when he struggled to remember. Sometimes he hesitated and searched for words; but he's intelligent and found alternatives to words he couldn't remember.

As for poor judgment, there was my nephew's accident at the Odessa intersection—the one that made me wonder and kept me awake.

The Alzheimer's Association booklet also lists ten symptoms of caregiver stress. Number one: *denial.* We deny the symptoms as long as we can because a future with Alzheimer's is too horrible to face.

My family was in denial about Dad for years. We laughed, for example, when he left ice cream in the hall closet instead of the freezer. But Mother stopped laughing a few years later when Dad forgot he parked the car in front of the bank and started walking home in the wrong direction.

I denied the severity of my father's condition when I asked him to help move my family from South Dakota to Indiana. I was lucky he made it home without killing someone.

Dad's generation, in turn, was in denial about my grandfather's condition. That's why they couldn't figure out what caused his accident at the Huntoon crossing, and why they attributed his later symptoms to grief.

But perhaps I was wrong to worry about my nephew. Maybe he was just a little more forgetful than the average fifty-year-old. When I had dinner with his family before our trip to the panhandle, we began reminiscing about the past. His worried wife asked him several times, "Do you remember that?" Her voice crackled with anxiety. In subtle ways she kept reminding him that he might have the Alzheimer's gene, that he was next in line. Maybe his forgetfulness wasn't stamped into his genetic coding. Maybe my nephew felt so pressured by his wife's reminders that he'd unconsciously adopted the symptoms.

I didn't blame my nephew's wife for applying pressure; I knew she was anxious (number four on the list of symptoms of caregiver stress) and she was on the verge of anger (number two) and depression (number five).

When my nephew's wife emailed me about his accident, she gave me another piece of news: they had a new grandson, their second, named Amos Nick. In my reply, I congratulated them and told her the baby's name made him sound part prophet and part gambler. I pressed the send key before I realized the full meaning of what I'd written.

Amos Nick is only one-sixteenth Volga German, a long way from the ethnic purity of my father's generation. Despite the mixture of blood in his veins, if his grandfather has the gene—and the accident in Odessa may be an indication that he does—Amos Nick has the same odds of getting early onset Alzheimer's disease as my siblings and I had when our grandfather drove the truck onto the Huntoon crossing. Amos Nick may become a skilled gambler, but even if he studies his cards and knows when to hold 'em and when to fold 'em, his parents already played his hand with a high-stakes gamble at conception.

A tremendous life force drives people to love, make love, have children. Young people in my family will continue to have babies, even if they are in line for the gene. Rita and I had our son, Jesse, before we know whether we'd be consigning him to the possibility of an early death and his family to the severest test of love anyone can endure.

Amos Nick's family has faith that things will be okay; if not, they'll manage with the help of God. But it's evident to me, at least, that prayer won't persuade God to solve genetic problems.

Much has changed in the seven decades between the accidents at the Huntoon crossing and the Odessa intersection. We've moved from ignorance to understanding. We know our family has a genetic affliction, early onset

Alzheimer's disease (EOAD in the scientific literature). With a drop of blood, science can tell each of us whether or not we will get the disease. Newly developed drugs may slow its progression. Worldwide, researchers are conducting hundreds of research projects and experiments to find preventions, treatments, and cures for EOAD and its later sporadic onset version. Hope soars.

Speaking before the Senate Committee on Aging, Dr. Tanzi of Harvard and Massachusetts General Hospital said that in five years we will have ways to treat and prevent the disease. We hope, we pray he is right. As I write these words, my family waits.

As for me, I won the genetic coin toss. I now look at the situation as an outsider. My children are free to find their own problems; early onset Alzheimer's won't haunt their lives. So why am I lying awake, filled with fear?

For one thing, it's an old habit to be afraid of this disease. I've been afraid since 1963 when doctors diagnosed Alzheimer's in my dad and told us the illness was probably hereditary. No, I was fearful even before that, when the first changes began to creep into my father's behavior. And even before that, when I took my ailing grandfather for walks sixty-five years ago and tried to keep him from touching the electric fences at our farm. And now I know, from the research done at the Univeristy of Washington, that I have one copy of Apo-E4, making the odds I will have Alzheimer's by age eighty, one decade from now, about fifty-fifty.

Having lived so long with the fear of this death, I sometimes feel detached from those who have not lived with it. I passionately hope my nephew's accident in Odessa was not caused by early symptoms of Alzheimer's. I hope his branch of the family wins the genetic coin toss for EOAD, as I did, so Amos Nick will be free to play his own hand. My impulse is to pray that it is so. So I sit here awake, and hope (and pray), and write, trying to calm my fear with words. As the last man standing, what else can I do?

*

As I neared completion of this book, I sent an email message to my relatives, updating them on its progress and inviting them to say anything they wanted about their experiences living with the legacy of Alzheimer's. After six or eight weeks, I received a message back from my nephew's wife.

Dear Gary,

I just found the courage to open up your email about the book. I cannot find the words, unusual for me, I know, but it is too much for me to think of (name omitted) and this disease. He is forgetting things that hit us in the pit of the stomach. I am trying, and he has an appointment for genetic counseling on the ninth, and we will see where it goes from there. . . . Right now, it is not pretty, as we look each other in the eye and just start weeping, knowing what is ahead and HATING every single thought of it.

Love and sorrow,
(name omitted by author)

A few days later, I received another note from my nephew's wife, more upbeat this time. Their daughter is expecting their third grandchild; they're hoping for a girl to go with their two boys. Once my nephew finishes his genetic counseling, they will send his blood to Dr. Bird in Seattle, who will tell them for sure if he has the gene.

Afterword

The morning after I made the final changes to the galley of this book and sent it back to the publisher, I received two pieces of news. An international team of scientists has identified two new genes, CLU on chromosome 8, and PICALM on chromosome 11, the first new genes found in more than a decade. These genes, in addition to ApoE4, the other gene besides PS2 that is prominent in my family, increase the risk of getting late onset Alzheimer's. Their discovery will help in the development of drugs for treatment and possibly a cure for Alzheimer's, both early onset and sporadic onset.

At the same time this hopeful news arrived, I received a note from my cousin, the younger son of Aunt Ester May and Uncle George. He was forming a group in the annual Memory Walk in his community to raise money for the Alzheimer's Association. He also informed those he was asking to contribute that he has early onset Alzheimer's. I was shocked. I hoped, to the extent that I believed, he had been skipped by the gene. While scientific advances bring optimism, the genetic anomaly in my family takes its toll

To live with these contradictions, all we can do is what we are doing. We participate in the Alzheimer's Association and other organizations that promote awareness, take part in research whenever there is an opportunity, and keep ourselves informed. This is not easy for our family. It requires the sacrifice of some personal privacy. And that sacrifice is especially difficult for a family in which personal privacy is a deep-rooted—even historic—need, one which dates back to our ancestors living in Russia, in a closed Volga German society, keeping to themselves in order to avoid taxes, military conscription, and other confrontations with the government. But with the leadership of Aunt Ester in the last generation and Chuck in this generation, more of us are stepping forward and speaking out.